Date: 6/22/18

617.1027 SPO
Sports injuries information
for teens : health tips about

Teen Health Series

Sports Injuries Information For Teens, Fourth Edition

Sports Injuries Information For Teens, Fourth Edition

Health Tips About Acute, Traumatic, And Chronic Injuries
In Adolescent Athletes

Including Facts About Sprains, Fractures, And Overuse Injuries,
Treatment, Rehabilitation, Sport-Specific Safety Guidelines, Fitness
Suggestions, And More

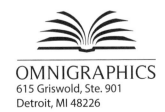

OMNIGRAPHICS
615 Griswold, Ste. 901
Detroit, MI 48226

Bibliographic Note
Because this page cannot legibly accommodate all the copyright notices, the Bibliographic Note portion of the Preface constitutes an extension of the copyright notice.

* * *

Omnigraphics
a part of Relevant Information
Siva Ganesh Maharaja, *Managing Editor*

* * *

Copyright © 2017 Omnigraphics
ISBN 978-0-7808-1567-4
E-ISBN 978-0-7808-1568-1

Library of Congress Cataloging-in-Publication Data

Names: Omnigraphics, Inc., issuing body.

Title: Sports injuries information for teens: health tips about acute, traumatic, and chronic injuries in adolescent athletes including facts about sprains, fractures, and overuse injuries, treatment, rehabilitation, sport-specific safety guidelines, fitness suggestions, and more.

Description: Fourth edition. | Detroit, MI: Omnigraphics, [2017] | Series: Teen health series | Audience: Grade 9 to 12. | Includes bibliographical references and index.

Identifiers: LCCN 2017029918 (print) | LCCN 2017030115 (ebook) | ISBN 9780780815681 (eBook) | ISBN 9780780815674 (hardcover: alk. paper)

Subjects: LCSH: Sports injuries. | Teenagers--Wounds and injuries--Prevention. | Wounds and injuries.

Classification: LCC RD97 (ebook) | LCC RD97.S689 2017 (print) | DDC 617.1/027--dc23

LC record available at https://lccn.loc.gov/2017029918

Table Of Contents

Preface

Part One: Health Tips For Student Athletes

Part Two: Sports Safety And Injury Prevention

Part Three: Diagnosing And Treating Common Sports Injuries

Part Four: Caring For Injured Athletes

Part Five: If You Need More Information

Preface

About This Book

Participating in sports is great for teens—physically, socially, and mentally, and according to the President's Council on Fitness, Sports & Nutrition (PCFSN), more than 44 million young people participate in organized sports in the United States. While sports participation is beneficial in many ways, it also carries risk. A recent study found that more than 2.6 million children and teens participating in sports will be injured, and one in four sports injuries is considered serious. By observing proper training practices and using appropriate protective gear, however, young athletes can help minimize the risks they face.

Sports Injuries Information For Teens, Fourth Edition offers teens a comprehensive, fact-based guide to being a healthy athlete. It includes guidelines for participating safely in sports and avoiding injury. It also discusses how to deal with injuries when they do occur. It explains diagnostic and treatment procedures and discusses issues related to rehabilitation, including suggestions for making decisions about returning to play. The book concludes with directories of resources for more information about sports-related injuries and fitness.

How To Use This Book

This book is divided into parts and chapters. Parts focus on broad areas of interest; chapters are devoted to single topics within a part.

Part One: Health Tips For Student Athletes focuses on the important choices sports participants make about healthy lifestyles. It discusses choosing the right sports, sports physicals, basic nutrition, emotional issues, and substance abuse among athletes.

Part Two: Sports Safety And Injury Prevention summarizes guidelines for achieving and maintaining a level of fitness necessary to help avoid injuries. It describes the proper use of important protective equipment, including various types of helmets and eye protectors This part also offers specific safety tips for many popular sports.

Part Three: Diagnosing And Treating Common Sports Injuries explains the differences between acute and chronic injuries, and it discusses problems associated with extreme heat conditions.

It also describes the symptoms, treatment, and management of injuries that may occur among athletes, including sprains, strains, broken bones, concussions, and other injuries to the body's musculoskeletal system and soft tissues.

Part Four: Caring For Injured Athletes offers facts about the rehabilitation process, beginning with immediate care during the first moments after injury. It describes the important role of athletic trainers in helping assess and prevent injuries, offers suggestions for choosing a doctor and making medical decisions, and provides tips for caring for casts and splints. Guidelines for returning to play are presented, and the part concludes with information about the connection between sports injuries and the potential for the later development of arthritis.

Part Five: If You Need More Information offers resource directories of organizations able to provide more information about traumatic and chronic sports-related injuries and fitness and exercise.

Bibliographic Note

This volume contains documents and excerpts from publications issued by the following government agencies: Agency for Healthcare Research and Quality (AHRQ); Centers for Disease Control and Prevention (CDC); *Eunice Kennedy Shriver* National Institute of Child Health and Human Development (NICHD); Federal Occupational Health (FOH); Genetics Home Reference (GHR); *Go4Life*; National Aeronautics and Space Administration (NASA); National Center for Complementary and Integrative Health (NCCIH); National Eye Institute (NEI); National Highway Traffic Safety Administration (NHTSA); National Institute of Arthritis and Musculoskeletal and Skin Diseases (NIAMS); National Institute on Alcohol Abuse and Alcoholism (NIAAA); National Institute on Drug Abuse (NIDA); National Institute on Drug Abuse (NIDA) for Teens; National Institutes of Health (NIH); Office of Dietary Supplements (ODS); Office of Disease Prevention and Health Promotion (ODPHP); Office on Women's Health (OWH); President's Council on Fitness, Sports & Nutrition (PCFSN); U.S. Bureau of Labor Statistics (BLS); U.S. Consumer Product Safety Commission (CPSC); U.S. Department of Agriculture (USDA); U.S. Department of Education (ED); U.S. Department of Health and Human Services (HHS); U.S. Department of Veterans Affairs (VA); and U.S. Public Health Service Commissioned Corps (PHSCC).

It may also contain original material produced by Omnigraphics and reviewed by medical consultants.

The photograph on the front cover is © Mixmike/iStock.

Medical Review

Omnigraphics contracts with a team of qualified, senior medical professionals who serve as medical consultants for the *Teen Health Series*. As necessary, medical consultants review reprinted and originally written material for currency and accuracy. Citations including the phrase, Reviewed (month, year)" indicate material reviewed by this team. Medical consultation services are provided to the *Teen Health Series* editors by:

Dr. Vijayalakshmi, MBBS, DGO, MD
Dr. Senthil Selvan, MBBS, DCH, MD
Dr. K. Sivanandham, MBBS, DCH, MS (Research), PhD

About The *Teen Health Series*

At the request of librarians serving today's young adults, the *Teen Health Series* was developed as a specially focused set of volumes within Omnigraphics' *Health Reference Series*. Each volume deals comprehensively with a topic selected according to the needs and interests of people in middle school and high school. Teens seeking preventive guidance, information about disease warning signs, medical statistics, and risk factors for health problems will find answers to their questions in the *Teen Health Series*. The *Series*, however, is not intended to serve as a tool for diagnosing illness, in prescribing treatments, or as a substitute for the physician/patient relationship. All people concerned about medical symptoms or the possibility of disease are encouraged to seek professional care from an appropriate healthcare provider.

If there is a topic you would like to see addressed in a future volume of the *Teen Health Series*, please write to:

Editor
Teen Health Series
Omnigraphics
615 Griswold, Ste. 901
Detroit, MI 48226

A Note About Spelling And Style

Teen Health Series editors use *Stedman's Medical Dictionary* as an authority for questions related to the spelling of medical terms and the *Chicago Manual of Style* for questions related to grammatical structures, punctuation, and other editorial concerns. Consistent adherence is not always possible, however, because the individual volumes within the *Series* include many documents from a wide variety of different producers and copyright holders, and the editor's primary goal is to present material from each source as accurately as is possible following the terms specified by each document's producer. This sometimes means that information in different chapters may follow other guidelines and alternate spelling authorities. For example, occasionally a copyright holder may require that eponymous terms be shown in possessive forms (Crohn's disease vs. Crohn disease) or that British spelling norms be retained (leukaemia vs. leukemia).

Part One
Health Tips For Student Athletes

Chapter 1

Choosing The Right Sport For You

Making Room For Sports

Sports can give a big boost to the amount of physical activity in your life. You can choose individual activities like: biking, running, swimming, or hiking. Or, you may want to celebrate your social—and perhaps more competitive—side by joining a team or a club. Research your local community to find adult teams to join such as: soccer, baseball, basketball, hockey, football, tennis, or even Ultimate Frisbee. You may also be able to catch a pick-up game at your local parks department or gym. You can find "meet-up" groups on the Internet for other sports enthusiasts in your area. There are also classes. This is a great way to introduce yourself to a new sport and skill set.

So, whatever activity or sports that you choose, remember to check with your physician first, and take care to slowly warm up your muscles and joints before you start any strenuous activity. Also, give yourself time to cool down and gently stretch when you're finished. And, most of all, pick something you truly enjoy and do it regularly.

Why Choose Sports?

Playing sports can help you make friends, boost your mood, and teach you tons of skills. Those who play sports may:

- Have greater self-esteem and less depression

About This Chapter: Text under the heading "Making Room For Sports" is excerpted from "Rise To The President's Challenge...Make Physical Activity Part Of Your Life," Federal Occupational Health (FOH), U.S. Department of Health and Human Services (HHS), May 1, 2014; Text beginning with the heading "Why Choose Sports?" is excerpted from "Playing Sports," girlshealth.gov, Office on Women's Health (OWH), March 27, 2015; Text under the heading, "Tips To Stay Fit On Campus" is excerpted from "10 Tips: Stay Fit On Campus," ChooseMyPlate.gov, U.S. Department of Agriculture (USDA), February 16, 2017.

- Learn how to set goals and work hard

- Have a more positive body image

- Learn about working as part of a team

- Do better in school

Picking A Sport

It helps to think about a few issues when choosing a sport. Start by asking yourself some questions:

- Do you like to work together with teammates, the way you do in soccer or lacrosse?

- Do you prefer to work more on your own, as in swimming or track?

- How do you feel about competition? Does it twist your tummy? Maybe inviting a friend to shoot hoops or go hiking is more for you.

- Do you like to keep moving? Does soccer, basketball, or field hockey sound fun to you?

- Do you like music? You might think about dance and cheerleading, which can offer great workouts.

- Are you interested in relaxing and connecting your mind and body, like you do in yoga or Pilates?

Safety In Sports

Stay in the game with these tips:

- **If you're new to a sport**, work your way up slowly.

- **Before you start a sport, see your doctor for a sports physical.** Some states require these examinations to make sure you are healthy enough to play. But even if a sports physical is not required, it makes good sense to get one.

- **Follow safety rules for your sport.** In cheerleading, for example, don't practice on hard, wet, or uneven surfaces, and don't create pyramids that are more than two people high. And learn what to do in case of an injury or emergency.

- **Talk to your coach about any safety concerns,** or ask your parent or guardian to talk to your coach.

- **Learn how to help your teammates stay safe.** For sports like cheerleading or gymnastics, for example, learn how to be a good spotter.

- **Make sure to read about concussions.** Anyone who might have a head injury should not practice or compete until a health professional says it's safe.

- **Give your body a break.** Experts suggest the following:

  - Take at least one day off per week from your sport or training schedule.

  - Take at least two to three months off from your sport each year.

  - If you train a lot in a high-impact sport, such as running, try replacing some intense training with lower-impact activities, such as biking.

- **Try different sports.** Playing the same sport over and over can put repeated stress on certain parts of your body. Doing a mix of sports and activities can help prevent this problem.

- **Strengthen your muscles.** Conditioning exercises, such as sit-ups and push-ups, can strengthen the muscles you use when you compete. Learn more about strengthening exercises.

- **Skip special supplements.** Products may claim to help you lose weight, bulk up, or improve your performance. Often these don't work, and they can even hurt you. Remember, all you really need to succeed is good nutrition

Tips To Stay Fit In Campus

Between classes and studying, it can be difficult to find time to be active. Even if you only exercise for a short period of time, you will feel more energized and better about your health. Get up and move!

1. **Walk or bike to class**

   If you live close enough to campus, avoid driving or spending money on public transportation by walking or biking to class. If you drive to campus, park your car farther away from the building to lengthen your walk.

2. **Take the stairs**

   As tempting as the elevators and escalators are, avoid them by using the stairs. This exercise is a great habit to start and will help tone your legs at the same time!

3. **Join a sport**

   Find a sport that interests you the most and one that will keep you active during your spare time. If you played a sport in high school such as basketball or soccer, you can continue playing in college!

4. **Join an intramural team**

   Another fun way to remain active is by joining an intramural team. Most universities offer classic sports such as basketball or baseball. But some campuses also offer activities such as ultimate frisbee and bowling.

5. **Hit the gym!**

   Visit your school's gym or recreation center. Go for a run on an indoor track or grab a basketball and shoot some hoops. Try to vary your routine each time to avoid boredom.

6. **Be active with friends**

   Go for a walk, hike, or bike ride with friends to catch up and have fun!

7. **Take a fitness class**

   Most universities offer a wide range of fitness classes for little or no charge. Find a schedule online and choose a class that you enjoy such as yoga, spinning, kickboxing, or aerobics.

8. **Fitness for credit**

   Elective classes such as swimming are a great way to remain active while also earning school credit. Not only are these classes fun, but they offer you a scheduled workout once or twice a week. Sign up with friends or try out a new class that strikes your interest.

9. **Sign up for an adventure trip**

   Many universities also offer adventure trips, such as hiking and whitewater rafting, to their students at a discounted price. Check out your university's recreation website for a list of upcoming events, and sign up for an active trip.

10. **Balance calories!**

   What you eat is just as important as how active you are. Keep track of how much you eat and your daily physical activity to help you to maintain a healthy weight.

Chapter 2

Sports For Students With Disabilities

Children and adolescents with disabilities are more likely to be inactive than those without disabilities. Youth with disabilities should work with their healthcare provider to understand the types and amounts of physical activity appropriate for them. When possible, children and adolescents with disabilities should meet the Guidelines. When young people are not able to participate in appropriate physical activities to meet the Guidelines, they should be as active as possible and avoid being inactive. In order to reduce the risk of injury, children and youth are advised to increase their physical activity gradually and to engage in a variety of exercise, sport, and recreation activities. Increased physical activity increases motor skills, which in turn facilitate increased physical activity.

Accessibility

Accessibility includes the considerations of the area or environment in which physical activity takes place, the safety and security within the space, and specifications suggested for particular disabilities. Access is facilitated through adapted PE (physical education) practices and universal design principles. For example, concrete play areas are being replaced by soft surfaces to reduce child injury. Because wood chips and sand interfere with mobility of children and youth in wheelchairs, solid soft surfaces are recommended to allow safe use of play areas by more children and youth.

About This Chapter: This chapter includes text excerpted from "Creating Equal Opportunities For Children And Youth With Disabilities To Participate In Physical Education And Extracurricular Athletics," U.S. Department of Education (ED), August 2011. Reviewed July 2017.

Equipment

Appropriate equipment can help children and youth with disabilities participate in appropriate physical activity. Athletic equipment might need to be modified for safe use by some children and youth with disabilities. For other students with disabilities, specialized equipment may be needed. Activities involving the use of modified or specialized equipment can replace other less safe activities. Treadmills, for example, are effective in providing predictable walking and running conditions, which can be necessary and appropriate for some individuals with disabilities. As another example, gaming systems that support movement detection technologies (e.g., Wii, Xbox 360, and PlayStation 3) can be used by some children and youth with disabilities to participate in sport simulations. Physical growth and development and changes in ability require continuous reevaluation and, as needed, modification of the fit and functionality of equipment for children and youth with disabilities

Personnel Preparation

Knowledgeable adults create the possibility of participation among children and youth both with and without disabilities. Physical activities may be guided by a wide range of support personnel with various levels of training including other students, general and special education teachers, paraprofessionals, adaptive physical education specialists, and related service providers (e.g., occupational therapist or speech language pathologist). Appropriate personnel preparation and professional development to adapt games and activities to various ability and fitness levels are needed in order to increase opportunities for children and youth with disabilities.

Teaching Style

Inclusive teaching styles create a climate and culture of participation for children and youth with and without disabilities. The educational philosophy and beliefs of the individual teacher and the school system influence opportunity. Patterns of teaching must be informed by the need to safeguard the civil rights of all students, including those with disabilities, both by providing equal athletic opportunity and protecting students from reasonably foreseeable risks to their health and safety. In PE and athletic programs, the focus has traditionally been on competition rather than instruction, but has recently shifted to "new PE," which focuses on improvements by the individual student. Children and youth with disabilities and those without athletic prowess require adaptive opportunities and precise instruction for concerns such as poor motor coordination.

Management Of Behavior

Athletics in the school setting involve complex interactions in settings less controlled than the typical academic classroom. Team play and sportsmanship cannot be taught except through participation. Effective PE and athletics require a teacher or coach with strong behavior management skills. Certain disabilities are associated with characteristics that may interfere with the student's ability to act consistently like a good team player or otherwise conform to the social expectations of particular athletic activities. A few of these characteristics include poor impulse control, limited social awareness, and emotional lability. School personnel should have the knowledge, skills, and abilities to address the interactional components of disabilities within the context of competition. Children and youth with and without disabilities can participate in PE and athletics more fully when social, emotional, and behavioral interactions are directly instructed, monitored, and remediated.

Program Options

PE and athletics can be offered in various degrees of inclusion in programs and activities with children and youth without disabilities. IDEA (Individuals with Disabilities Education Act) requires that each child with a disability participates with nondisabled children in these programs and activities to the maximum extent appropriate to the needs of that child. Physical education services, specially designed if necessary, must be made available to every child with a disability receiving a free appropriate public education, unless the public agency enrolls children without disabilities and does not provide physical education to children without disabilities in the same grades. Each public agency must take steps to provide nonacademic and extracurricular services and activities, including athletics, in the manner necessary to afford children with disabilities an equal opportunity for participation in those services and activities. For students served under IDEA, the student's IEP (Individualized Education Program) must include, among other things, a statement of the special education and related services, and supplementary aids, services, and other supports that are needed to meet each child's unique needs in order for the child to:

1. advance appropriately towards attaining the annual goals;

2. be involved in and make progress in the general education curriculum and to participate in extracurricular and other nonacademic activities; and

3. be educated and participate in such activities with other children with disabilities and nondisabled children.

The IEP team, which includes both general and special education teachers, might benefit from participation by a general or adaptive physical education teacher in order to develop the IEP for certain students.

Curriculum

Curriculum encompasses more than the age or grade lists of content standards, benchmarks, objectives, strategies, and assessments. Curriculum includes day-to-day implementation, which requires flexibility with the content in context. An accessible PE curriculum provides for that flexibility. Applying the universal design for learning (UDL) framework to the PE curriculum increases opportunities for participation by providing multiple means for student engagement. The variety of options allows children with disabilities to choose activities of interest which increases their participation. UDL also provides multiple means of presentation. Information technology shows promise in providing a new means of presentation.

For example, "bug-in-the-ear" communicators allow sideline coaches and instructors to personalize the "real-time" explanation of game rules and procedures based on the needs of individual players with disabilities. PE curricula based on physical growth and the development of fitness and socialization can support the inclusion of children and youth with disabilities. The curricular focus on lifelong fitness and health can facilitate forming habits that will follow through to adulthood. Teachers and coaches increase successful inclusion by focusing on the camaraderie and fun of activity rather than on competition and winning. An individual student's IEP must include goals and accommodations for PE and athletics, as needed. The development of IEPs requires collaboration among professionals as well as parent participation. Parents might be reluctant to have their children participate in physical activity due to uncertainty about its effects and the possibility of teasing and ridicule from peers. The IEP team can better support the students' successful access to, and participation in, PE and athletics when these concerns are effectively addressed in the IEP.

Assessment, Progress, Achievement, And Grading

Assessment in PE and athletics should be planned and implemented so that progress and achievement can be rated accurately and fairly. Assessment instruments that compare the individual against herself or himself are able to measure both attainment and growth. These comparisons show the trajectory toward health and fitness, while avoiding the inappropriate application of some standardized benchmarks of health and fitness to children and youth with disabilities.

For example, body mass index (BMI) has been shown to be inappropriate for people with certain disabilities who tend to have a different proportion of lean mass. Some equipment and technologies may allow for more accurate assessments of the incremental improvements made by children and youth with disabilities. For instance, wheelchair scales increase the accurate measurement of a student's weight and a spreadsheet can track the changes. Better assessment can lead to better instruction, feedback, grading practices, and ultimately better outcomes for children and youth with disabilities. When competitive performance is the sole or primary criterion for grades in PE classes, some children and youth with and without disabilities might earn failing grades. The methods used to grade progress and achievement can be used to encourage participation among children and youth with disabilities. For an individual child whose IEP includes annual goals for PE and athletics, the IEP must include a description of how a child's progress towards meeting the annual goals will be measured.

Chapter 3

Sports Physicals

What Is A Sports Physical?

A sports physical exam, also known as preparticipation physical examination (PPE), is a medical evaluation used to determine if it is safe for you to play specific sports in school. In the United Sates, millions of teens undergo sports physicals before being cleared for competitive sports. A sports physical is different from a standard medical checkup. In a sports physical, a medical practitioner reviews past medical history and looks for diseases, injuries, and other factors that could impact a student athlete's performance or prevent them from participating at all.

Why Are Sports Physicals Essential?

Sports are a great way to stay fit and socialize with other kids of the same age. Most kids are anxious to get onto the field and start playing rather than being bothered with a medical evaluation. Rough and tumble is common in sports and there is a constant risk of injury. However, prevention is an essential aspect of staying safe on the field, and sports physicals help teens keep from getting hurt, injured, or becoming sick during competition. Sports physicals help identify high risk conditions that could compromise a teen's ability to play. Existing injuries, underlying disorders, and potential defects can be identified and accounted for early on. Sports physicals confirm that teens are in shape and ready for the season.

"Sports Physicals," © 2017 Omnigraphics. Reviewed July 2017.

When And Where Is A Sports Physical Done?

Sports physicals should occur around six to eight weeks before the beginning of sports season. Doing so allows young athletes time to recover from an existing injury or consult medical specialists before being cleared to play.

Teens and their parents can consult their pediatrician for a sports physical but most exams take place in schools, which often schedule on-site exam days with medical practitioners before the start of the season. In some states having a sports physical is mandatory and examinations could begin from the seventh grade. Even if a sports physical is not compulsory, it makes sense to have a personal physical exam. A sports physical is recommended once a year and, if you are healing from an injury, make sure a medical professional clears you to play. Having a sports physical at the start of sports season is not advisable in any case.

What Are The Goals And Objectives Of A Sports Physical?

A sports physical is done with the following goals and objectives in mind:

- Determine if the teen is in good health

- Evaluate current fitness levels

- Discover conditions that may predispose the teen to new injuries

- Assess existing injuries

- Identify underlying genetic factors that could increase risk of injury

- Assess the teen's current physical conditioning

What Happens During A Sports Physical?

A sports physical consists of two parts. The doctor reviews your medical history and completes a physical examination.

When a doctor reviews your medical history, he or she will want to know about past hospitalizations, injuries sustained, and existing medical conditions. The doctor will also seek information regarding the issues listed below:

- Hereditary diseases or serious illnesses in the family

- Illnesses when you were young such as asthma, epilepsy, or diabetes

- Immunizations (ones taken and needed)
- Excessive weight gain or loss in the past that is indicative of eating disorders
- Allergies
- Dental problems
- Vision, speech, and hearing problems
- Details of injuries sustained in the past such as sprains, fractures, or concussions
- Details of menstrual health
- Use of alcohol and drugs
- Episodes of fatigue, dizziness, and fainting
- Daily medications, including over-the-counter drugs, prescription drugs, and supplements

You will be asked to fill a questionnaire with details from your medical history. Do not guess the answers and provide answers thoughtfully. You can bring the form home and consult with your parents about your family medical history before answering the questionnaire. This is important because doctors are good at detecting possible conditions by examining patterns of family illnesses.

A physical examination focuses on the following areas:

- Height and weight
- Blood pressure
- Pulse rate
- Vision and hearing
- Heart and lung function
- Abdomen, ears, nose, and throat
- Cholesterol, hemoglobin count, and urinalysis
- Neurological reflexes and coordination
- Strength, flexibility, and mobility

The physical examination will include an evaluation of musculoskeletal issues such as spinal alignment, joints, posture, gait, range of motion, knee extension, and arm and leg function. Flexibility and endurance tests might also be conducted with the assistance of a coach or athletic trainer.

Once both evaluations are complete, the doctor fills out and signs a form if you are cleared to participate. Otherwise, the doctor may recommend further tests, treatment for medical conditions, or referral to a specialist.

What Happens After A Sports Physical?

Most student athletes are cleared to participate after a sports physical. However, if you are not, this does not in any way indicate the end of the road for you. Tests or follow-up exams could be as simple as checking your blood pressure after a few days. Or, for example, as an athlete, you might be experiencing knee pain every time you run. This could be the result of poor running technique, a knee injury in the past, or as simple as wearing shoes that are unsuitable. An orthopedist or sports medicine specialist can help you identify the situation and resolve it successfully.

It is highly unlikely that you will be asked to refrain from participating in sports. The goal of conducting a sports physical is to ensure that you stay safe on the field and not to prevent you from playing. Specialists will do their best to get you on the field.

References

1. "Sports Physicals," The Nemours Foundation, July 2016.
2. "Sports Physicals," Cleveland Clinic, 2017.
3. Saglimbeni, Anthony J, MD. "Sports Physicals," WebMD LLC., December 3, 2015.
4. Alli, Renee A., MD. "Physical Exams And Teen Sports," WebMD LLC., September 6, 2016.

Chapter 4

Nutrition For Student Athletes

Healthy Foods And Beverages For Youth In Sports

Nutritious eating habits promote healthy development and allow young people to perform their best in school and other activities. Youth sports are terrific venues for promoting health because sports touch the lives of many youth. Today, youth sports are more popular than they have ever been. More than 44 million youth in the United States participate in sports each year, and two in three students in high school play on at least one sports team at their school or in their community. Sports, including soccer, basketball, tennis, and dance, among others, offer youth an opportunity to engage in vigorous physical activity while they learn how to work together, have fun, and compete toward a common goal. For these reasons and many more, participation in sport can promote healthy development for youth and adolescents.

Unhealthy Eating Is An Accepted Part Of Youth Sports

Unfortunately, youth sport activities are not currently living up to their potential as a setting for promoting healthy eating. According to the *Dietary Guidelines for Americans*, healthy eating emphasizes foods such as fruits, vegetables, whole grains, lean meats, and low-fat milk products. Healthy eating provides a balance of protein, carbohydrates, fat, water, vitamins, and minerals and a limited amount of calories. Unhealthy eating includes foods

About This Chapter: This chapter includes text excerpted from "Healthy Foods And Beverages For Youth In Sports," President's Council on Fitness, Sports & Nutrition (PCFSN), May 13, 2016.

and beverages that are high in fat, sugar, sodium, and calories. It is possible for youth to find unhealthy food and beverage options most anywhere they go, including from vending machines, concessions, convenience stores, and fast food restaurants. This is especially true in youth sport settings.

Youth who participate in sports consume more fast food, more sugary drinks, and more calories overall than youth who are not involved in sport. The foods and beverages that are convenient and widely available to youth in sport settings are generally unhealthy. For example, concession stands are common in youth sport settings. Typical choices at concession stands include items such as chocolate and other candy, ice cream, salty snacks, sugary beverages, and high-fat, calorie-dense entrees such as hot dogs and pizza. Healthier alternatives are rare. Additionally, parents often organize schedules for providing treats after each game for their child's team. These treats often include candy, doughnuts, chips, and sugary drinks. Parents report that team members and other parents can have a negative reaction when offering healthy choices for postevent treats, such as fruit. Youth sport schedules often overlap with regular family mealtimes and encourage eating away from home. Eating meals outside the home at fast food restaurants is associated with excess body weight and indicators of poor cardiovascular health.

Physical Activity And Eating Habits In Sport Are Out Of Balance

The widespread availability of unhealthy foods and beverages in sport settings helps contribute to a cultural norm of accepting, and even expecting, unhealthy eating as a part of youth sport. Parents and coaches view postgame snacks, concession stand items, and fast food meals in youth sport as an occasional indulgence that is permitted, even if it is inconsistent with the foods prepared at home. We have heard anecdotally, and when conducting systematic focus group research, that part of the reason that coaches and parents may relax their usual standards for healthy eating is that they see youth engaging in vigorous exercise during sport. Parents and coaches report that they believe this activity offsets the potential downside of any unhealthy foods or beverages they may have consumed. A common view of postgame treats is exemplified by the following statement from the parent of a child participating in sport: "These kids have been running around for an hour. They can have ice cream."

Despite this belief, research suggests that parents, coaches, and young athletes may overestimate the amount of physical activity sports provide. Studies that objectively measure the amount of physical activity youth gain during sports have found that only about one in four achieve recommended levels of daily activity. The U.S. Department of Health and Human Services (HHS) *Physical Activity Guidelines for Americans* recommend that children and adolescents accumulate 60 minutes of moderate to vigorous physical activity each day. Examples of moderate intensity physical activity for adolescents include baseball, yard work, hiking, and brisk walking while examples of vigorous activity include jumping rope, bike riding, karate, basketball, and cross-country skiing. The objective evidence suggests that participating in sports provides an average of 30 minutes of the recommended 60 minutes of physical activity. While most sports involve vigorous physical activity, they also involve considerable time in light activity or no activity, such as waiting on the sidelines to enter the game and standing around between plays or while receiving instruction from coaches. The amount of energy expended in sport can vary by type of sport, age of the participant, coaching practices, and other factors, but the data suggest the amount of energy expended in sports is relatively modest. If youth consume the types of foods that are widely available in youth sport settings, they may be overcompensating for the amount of energy they expended in the sport's activity by taking in extra calories. They are also consuming foods and beverages that may fail to provide the appropriate balance of nutrients that comprise a healthy diet.

Why Is Healthy Eating So Challenging For Young Athletes?

Recent research has started to identify some of the challenges to healthy eating for youth involved in sports. A significant contributor to the lack of healthy eating in youth sports is simply the busy schedules that many families with young children confront. Youth sport practices and competitions occur on several occasions each week at night, and on weekends. In some cases these events can entail considerable travel. Families with multiple children involved in sport and other activities can feel stretched thin simply from transporting them to various locations. Parents who participated in a research told that youth sport activities reduce the frequency of family meals at home. Parents and youth involved in activities want foods and beverages that are convenient and easy to consume while they are "on the go." The time pressures of their children's activities regularly lead them to pick up fast food and eat in the car on the way to or from youth sport events. Youth who attend sport competitions that involve several games or events over the course of a day often rely on foods and beverages from the concession stand.

Normative attitudes and behaviors also contribute to unhealthy eating in youth sport settings. Widespread availability of unhealthy foods and beverages makes them appear to be acceptable and expected.

In addition, teams will often have a postgame treat or meal at a fast food restaurant. Parents and coaches reported that the social benefits for the team (e.g., team bonding) often outweigh the importance of eating a more nutritious meal. Parents who are committed to good nutrition can find it difficult to voice their concerns in these situations. Finally, parents and coaches of teams reported that they did not feel they had adequate knowledge about nutrition and the best ways to properly feed young athletes. Participants in a research reported that they were sometimes confused by seemingly conflicting advice about nutrition in the media and they wanted clear guidance about what was best for youth involved in sports.

Table 4.1. Estimated Calorie Needs Per Day By Age, Gender, And Physical Activity Level

Age (Years)	Males			Females		
	Sedentary	Moderately Active	Active	Sedentary	Moderately Active	Active
9–13	1,600–2,000	1,800–2,200	2,000–2,600	1,400–1,600	1,600–2,000	1,800–2,200
14–16	2,000–2,400	2,400–2,800	2,800–3,200	1,800	2,000	2,400
17–18	2,400	2,800	3,200	1,800	2,000	2,400

What Does A Developing Young Athlete Need To Eat?

Despite the many challenges, youth who participate in sports can benefit from eating a well-balanced, nutritious diet. In general, the dietary needs of youth athletes do not significantly differ from their nonsport participating counterparts. The *Dietary Guidelines for Americans 2015–2020* recommend a balanced intake that consists of fruits and vegetables, grains (with at least half whole grains), fat-free or low-fat dairy, a variety of protein foods, and oils. Also recommended is limiting the amount of saturated fat, added sugars, and sodium (salt). Consuming a variety of these foods provides adequate macronutrients and micronutrients needed to support youth development and optimal sport performance. Macronutrients are nutrients the body needs in larger amounts (e.g., carbohydrate, protein, and fat) and micronutrients are nutrients the body needs in smaller amounts (e.g., vitamins and minerals). Each macro- and micro-nutrient plays an essential role in healthy youth development. The roles macronutrients play in the body and food sources of each are described below.

Carbohydrate: Carbohydrate is the main fuel source for the body. Once digested, the body converts carbohydrate to glucose that will be used for energy or stored for later use in the muscles and liver. There are two types of carbohydrate: simple and complex. Simple carbohydrates are digested more quickly and are found in fruit, vegetables, and dairy. Complex carbohydrates are digested more slowly and are found in a variety of foods including bread, pasta, and rice.

Sources: Whole grains (pasta, bread, rice), dairy, fruit, vegetables

Protein: Protein helps regulate the function of cells, tissues, and organs in the body. For athletes, protein is also important for muscle repair and recovery.

Sources: Lean meat and poultry, fish, beans, dairy, eggs, nuts/seeds

Fat: Fat provides energy when carbohydrate is not available, is essential for the absorption of some vitamins (A, D, E, and K), and aids in maintaining body temperature.

Sources: Oil, avocado, nuts/seeds

How Many Daily Calories Does A Youth Athlete Need?

Nutritional needs for athletes depend on many factors including age, gender, sport, and activity/competition level. Depending on activity intensity (e.g., sedentary, moderate or vigorous intensity), different daily calorie needs are recommended for youth by the U.S. Department of Agriculture (USDA) and U.S. Department of Health and Human Services (HHS). Examples of moderate intensity activities include riding a bike and walking briskly. Vigorous (i.e., active) activities include running, jumping rope, and playing sports such as basketball, soccer, tennis, and hockey. These activities should make youth sweat and breathe hard. The calorie recommendations based on different activity levels for males and females are shown in Table 4.1. Finding the right balance between energy expenditure and energy intake will help an athlete avoid energy deficit or excess. Energy deficit can delay growth and puberty, as well as impact bone density, and energy excess can lead to overweight.

Eating Before An Activity/Sport

For youth involved in sport, eating before an activity is essential to provide the body with enough energy for best performance. For activities that are in the morning, eat breakfast at least one hour in advance. Finding a good combination of complex and simple carbohydrates with some protein and fat, such as a piece of whole wheat toast (complex carbohydrate) with peanut butter (protein and fat) and a small banana (simple carbohydrate), will provide a slow release of energy throughout the activity. For activities that occur after school, athletes could benefit from eating a snack about an hour before the activity to allow enough digestion time to prevent stomach discomfort during the activity. Some individuals may experience discomfort from meals/snacks that are higher in fat and fiber before activity. A combination of carbohydrates, lower fat, lower fiber, and plenty of plain water may be ideal.

Some small meal examples may include yogurt with fruit, an apple with peanut butter, or whole grain crackers and string cheese. There are a variety of nutritious food options for young athletes to eat before an activity. Parents and coaches can work with their athletes to ensure that a balanced preactivity meal is consumed by the athlete prior to sport participation.

Eating During An Activity/Sport

Many youth athletes compete in all-day tournaments or have several games in one day. In this case, eating and hydrating between activities is important to fuel the body for the rest of the event. Eating five to six small meals throughout the day could be a good approach. These meals can consist of a variety of easy to digest, nutrient-dense ingredients that provide sustainable energy for the athletes to support their nutritional needs throughout the competition. When events are less than two hours apart, a nutrient-dense, high-carbohydrate snack like fruit with yogurt or a granola bar is ideal. A regular meal (e.g., whole wheat sandwich with lean meat and vegetables, a piece of fruit, and milk) can be eaten when games are longer than a few hours apart.

Eating After An Activity/Sport

Consuming carbohydrate- and protein-containing foods within a couple of hours postactivity can help to replenish energy stores that were used to fuel the activity and repair muscles. Parents, coaches, and young athletes should aim for whole foods (i.e., less processed) and foods that are bright and colorful (e.g., fruits and vegetables), such as whole wheat spaghetti with tomato sauce, chicken breast, a salad with a variety of vegetables, and milk.

Should Young Athletes Consume More Of Some Nutrients?

Overall, a well-balanced diet with plenty of water is adequate for youth who participate in sport. However, assuring athletes consume adequate amounts of calcium, vitamin D, and iron should be considered. Calcium supports muscle contraction, bone growth, and strength. The Recommended Dietary Allowance (RDA) for calcium is 1,300 mg/day for 9–18 year olds. Calcium-rich foods include dairy products, dark leafy green vegetables, and fortified cereals. Vitamin D is also essential for bone health and aids in calcium absorption. The Recommended Dietary Allowance for vitamin D is 600 IU/day for 6–18 year olds. Vitamin D-rich foods include egg yolks, tuna, fortified milk, orange juice, and cereals. Iron helps with muscle repair and improves the body's ability to transfer oxygen to working muscles. The Recommended Dietary Allowance for iron is 10 mg/day for 6–8 year olds, 8 mg/day for 9–13 year olds, 11 mg/day for 14–18 year old males and 15 mg/day for 14–18 year old females. Iron-rich foods include meat, poultry, beans, dark green vegetables, and iron-fortified cereals.

Is There Anything Athletes Should Limit?

The body's ability to perform will be enhanced if an athlete limits foods that are high in saturated fat, added sugars, and sodium. This includes fast food, processed foods, sweetened beverages (nondiet soft drinks/sodas, sweetened teas, flavored juice drinks, energy drinks, etc.), and snacks and beverages with added sugar. Unfortunately, these characteristics describe the foods and beverages that are typically available in youth sport settings. Not only could these foods and beverages inhibit athletic performance, but they can increase body weight and promote chronic disease. Youth involved in sports should choose foods that will fuel their body healthfully and provide sustainable nutrition for their needs as they compete.

Finding The Right Balance

Many parents believe their child needs a lot of additional calories because they are being physically active in sport. As noted in Table 4.1, however, active youth do not require considerably more calories than their peers who are less active. Young athletes (less than 12 years old) rarely burn enough energy (calories) through sport to require a supplemental snack. The additional calories may leave them vulnerable to excess weight gain. In recent years, it has become common for parents to provide snacks after games and practices. These snack foods are often high in calories and low in nutrients. Parents have a unique and important role when it comes to providing foods for their young athlete because parents are the primary influencer at this age.

Providing water and nutrient-dense snacks should be the focus, not "treats." As young athletes turn into adolescents, the primary influencer often shifts from parents to coaches and peers. Educating coaches, parents, and young athletes about proper fuel for enhanced performance is essential to reduce the likelihood of calorie overcompensation; that is, consuming too many calories post-game/practice than expended (burned). Parents and coaches may need additional education about the amount of calories and the right balance of foods their young athletes need. Unless a child is an endurance athlete or participating in an all-day event, three well-balanced meals that meet their caloric and nutrient needs, and possibly light nutritious snacks between meals, should supply sufficient energy.

Providing A Healthy Food Environment

A healthy food environment is one that provides nutritious foods and beverages that are affordable, convenient, and accessible in a way that makes them an easy choice. It also limits access to foods and beverages that have high levels of fat, sugar, sodium, and calories. The food environment at most youth sporting events is not very healthy. On game days, concession stands are stocked with high calorie, high sugar, and low nutrient foods such as hot dogs, pizza, "walking tacos," candy, and sodas/soft drink. The culture of concession stands has been to raise money for the hosting organization, as foods commonly served are high in demand and low in cost to prepare and/or offer. Parents also routinely provide post-game snacks that are sugary, salty, or fatty, rather than nutritious. Fast food restaurants are a convenient choice for busy families shuttling their children to various activities, including sport practices and events, but these venues tend to offer foods and beverages that are unhealthy.

Not only are these foods commonly available in youth sport settings undesirable for athletic performance, but some parents have expressed their concerns over the lack of available healthy options during sport events. Barriers to including healthful foods at sporting events include lack of sport nutrition knowledge and resistance to change because organizations rely on them for fund raising. Public health professionals are working with key stakeholders to improve the food environment in the home, in schools, at worksites, in child care centers, and in healthcare facilities. A similar focus is needed to improve the food environment in youth sport settings. Concerted effort is needed to improve the quality and offer more fresh, local, and healthy food and beverage options, provide appropriate portion sizes to meet the nutritional needs of young athletes, and support those settings by implementing and enforcing strong standards.

Sports are a fun and engaging opportunity for children and adolescents to develop healthy habits they can carry with them into adulthood. One of those skills can be healthy eating. However, the way youth sports are currently operating may be teaching youth and families unhealthy eating habits. Change is needed to support healthy, growing, youth athletes. More attention is needed to change the types of foods and beverages that are available and accepted in youth sport settings. Youth, parents, and coaches can become more aware of the unhealthy options that are available and speak out to make their preferences known. Parents can help organizations offer healthier options and figure out ways to make those options feasible and sustainable and align with fund raising goals. Organizations can commit to promoting health as a priority. Considerable change has occurred to improve the foods and beverages available in schools with the attention, commitment, and leadership of many different stakeholders. Similar change is needed, and is possible, for youth sport.

Chapter 5

Water And Nutrition For Athletes

Water Consumption

Getting enough water every day is important for your health. Healthy people meet their fluid needs by drinking when thirsty and drinking with meals. Most of your fluid needs are met through the water and beverages you drink. However, you can get some fluids through the foods that you eat. For example, broth soups and foods with high water content such as celery, tomatoes, or melons can contribute to fluid intake.

Dehydration can affect athletic performance and increase the risk of a medical emergency. During athletic events or physical activities, athletes must drink sufficient amounts of liquids to prevent dehydration. Athletes who know the importance of hydration are more likely to consume the needed amount of liquid. However, athletes are not the only ones who are at risk. Children enjoying outdoor activities are also at risk of suffering from dehydration.

(Source: "Hydration Station," National Aeronautics and Space Administration (NASA).)

Water Helps Your Body

- Keep your temperature normal
- Lubricate and cushion joints

About This Chapter: Text under the heading "Water Consumption" is excerpted from "Drinking Water—Water And Nutrition," Centers for Disease Control and Prevention (CDC), October 5, 2016; Text under the heading "Water Is The Best Choice" is excerpted from "Healthy Foods And Beverages For Youth In Sports," President's Council on Fitness, Sports & Nutrition (PCFSN), May 13, 2016.

- Protect your spinal cord and other sensitive tissues

- Get rid of wastes through urination, perspiration, and bowel movements

Your Body Needs More Water When You Are

- In hot climates

- More physically active

- Running a fever

- Having diarrhea or vomiting

If You Think You Are Not Getting Enough Water, These Tips May Help

- Carry a water bottle for easy access when you are at work of running errands.

- Freeze some freezer safe water bottles. Take one with you for ice-cold water all day long.

- Choose water instead of sugar-sweetened beverages. This can also help with weight management. Substituting water for one 20-ounce sugar sweetened soda will save you about 240 calories. For example, during the school day students should have access to drinking water, giving them a healthy alternative to sugar-sweetened beverages.

- Choose water when eating out. Generally, you will save money and reduce calories.

- Add a wedge of lime or lemon to your water. This can help improve the taste and help you drink more water than you usually do.

Water Is The Best Choice

Just like eating the right foods, athletes need to stay hydrated. Drinking fluids before, during, and after activity and sport will prevent dehydration and improve performance and recovery. Athletes should never be thirsty and plain, nonflavored water should always be the first choice. Drinking water is crucial to avoid dehydration in young athletes. A few signs of dehydration include thirst, decreased urine output, dark yellow-colored urine, dry mouth, headaches, irritability, dizziness, and weakness. In addition to preventing dehydration by replacing fluids that have been lost through sweat, water helps with digestion and regulates body temperature. The American Academy of Pediatrics (AAP) recommends athletes be adequately hydrated preactivity and continue to hydrate during and after activity.

Table 5.1. Amount Of Water Recommended Before, During, And After
Activity

Before Activity	Drink 2–3 cups (16–24 ounces) of water two to three hours before activity
During Activity	Up to 4–6 cups (~34–50 ounces) per hour of water for adolescent athletes and those who sweat excessively.
After Activity	Drink 2–3 cups (16–24 ounces) of water after activity for every pound of body weight lost.

Chapter 6

Sports And Energy Drinks

Energy drinks are widely promoted as products that increase alertness and enhance physical and mental performance. Marketing targeted at young people has been quite effective. Next to multivitamins, energy drinks are the most popular dietary supplement consumed by American teens and young adults. Almost one-third of teens between 12 and 17 years drink them regularly.

Caffeine is the major ingredient in most energy drinks—a 24-oz energy drink may contain as much as 500 mg of caffeine (similar to that in four or five cups of coffee). Energy drinks also may contain guarana (another source of caffeine sometimes called Brazilian cocoa), sugars, taurine, ginseng, B vitamins, glucuronolactone, yohimbe, carnitine, and bitter orange.

How Much Caffeine Is Okay?

The American Academy of Pediatrics (AAP) recommends that adolescents aged 12–18 years should not exceed 100 mg of caffeine a day, this is the amount of caffeine in a cup of coffee.

(Source: "The Buzz On Energy Drinks," Centers for Disease Control and Prevention (CDC).)

Consuming energy drinks also increases important safety concerns. A growing trend among young adults and teens is mixing energy drinks with alcohol. About 25 percent of college students consume alcohol with energy drinks, and they binge-drink significantly more often than students who don't mix them.

About This Chapter: This chapter includes text excerpted from "Energy Drinks," National Center for Complementary and Integrative Health (NCCIH), December 16, 2016.

Fast Facts

- While nationally only 1.2 percent of high schools sell energy drinks a la carte to students in the cafeteria, as many as 11.6 percent of secondary schools in some districts sell energy drinks in vending machines, school stores, and snack bars.
- Nationwide, 75 percent of school districts do not have a policy in place regarding these types of beverages that contain high levels of caffeine for sale in vending machines, schools stores, or a la carte in the cafeteria.

(Source: "The Buzz On Energy Drinks," Centers for Disease Control and Prevention (CDC).)

In 2011, 42 percent of all energy-drink related emergency department visits involved combining these beverages with alcohol or drugs (including illicit drugs, like marijuana, as well as central nervous system stimulants, like Ritalin or Adderall).

Bottom Line

- Although there's very limited data that caffeine-containing energy drinks may temporarily improve alertness and physical endurance, evidence that they enhance strength or power is lacking. More important, they can be dangerous because large amounts of caffeine may cause serious heart rhythm, blood flow, and blood pressure problems.

- There's not enough evidence to determine the effects of additives other than caffeine in energy drinks.

- The amounts of caffeine in energy drinks vary widely, and the actual caffeine content may not be identified easily.

Safety

- Large amounts of caffeine may cause serious heart and blood vessel problems such as heart rhythm disturbances and increases in heart rate and blood pressure. Caffeine also may harm children's still-developing cardiovascular and nervous systems.

- Caffeine use may be associated with palpitations, anxiety, sleep problems, digestive problems, elevated blood pressure, and dehydration.

- Guarana, commonly added to energy drinks, contains caffeine. Therefore, the addition of guarana increases the drink's total caffeine content.

- Young adults who combine caffeinated drinks with alcohol may not be able to tell how intoxicated they are.

- Excessive energy drink consumption may disrupt teens' sleep patterns and may fuel risk-taking behavior.

- Many energy drinks contain as much as 25–50 g of simple sugars; this may be problematic for people who are diabetic or prediabetic.

Energy Drink Recommendations For Adolescents

- The American Academy of Pediatrics (AAP) recommends that adolescents do not consume energy drinks, yet between 30–50 percent reported consuming energy drinks.
- The National Federation of State High School Associations (NFHS) recommends that young athletes should not use energy drinks for hydration, and information about the potential risk should be widely distributed to young athletes.

(Source: "The Buzz On Energy Drinks," Centers for Disease Control and Prevention (CDC).)

Chapter 7

Handling Sports Pressure And Competition

Negative Outcomes Of Sport Participation

While the research examining the link between sports participation and psychological and social outcomes is predominately positive, not all results have been favorable. For example, research has shown that certain athletes (e.g., those characterized as having high trait anxiety, low perceived competence), when placed in particular situations (e.g., situations where winning is perceived as highly important, event outcomes are very important), experience heightened levels of stress and may even experience burnout and motivational losses.

Factors Influencing Sport Participation And Social And Psychological Outcomes

Two context factors that have been found to influence the beneficial effects of sports participation on social and psychological outcomes are the motivational and caring climates created in the programs. Relative to the motivational climate, the more the climate is task- (focuses on self-improvement) versus ego-involving (focuses on comparison with others), provides autonomy of choice, and enhances enjoyment and positive adult peer relationships, the more likely positive outcomes will result. Over-emphasizing winning, employing authoritarian and harsh coaching practices, and engaging in constant social comparison have not been shown to be conducive to the development of social and emotional skills. Creating a caring program

About This Chapter: Text beginning with the heading "Negative Outcomes Of Sport Participation" is excerpted from "Elevate Health—Fitness—Sports—Nutrition," President's Council on Fitness, Sports & Nutrition (PCFSN), 2014; Text under the heading "Managing Stress In Sports" is excerpted from "Your Feelings—Feeling Stressed," girlshealth.gov, Office on Women's Health (OWH), April 1, 2015.

climate has also been shown to influence the outcomes of sports participation such as self-efficacy and social behaviors. Specifically, a caring climate is one where "each" participant is treated in a caring and supportive manner. Here, clear expectations relative to the team climate are widely understood by all participants and efforts are made to facilitate positive relationships between all involved.

Role Of Coaches And Sports Parents

The influence of the coach on social and psychological development of the athlete has been the focus of attention for a number of researchers. Results reveal that young athletes who play for coaches who have received training to be more encouraging and supportive in their orientation (versus those who have not) are characterized by a number of positive psychosocial outcomes. These include higher motivation for future involvement, decreased anxiety, increased enjoyment, and enhanced self-esteem. Other studies have shown that young athletes derive more benefits from sports participation if their coaches have philosophies that place importance on the development of socio-emotional life skills in their athletes. More effective coaches also establish trusting relationships with their athletes, intentionally teach life skills and emphasize psychosocial values and skills, spend more time teaching skills like goal setting, help their athletes establish competition strategies, and regularly talk about how sports lessons relate to life.

In addition to coaches, sports parents have been shown to have important influence on their child's youth sports experience. They also serve as role models who provide information about sports involvement, its importance, and how to interact with those in sports. Finally, parents serve as interpreters of their child's sports experience by influencing factors such as perceptions of competence and stress levels. For example, it was found that field hockey players who perceived that their parents placed greater importance on doing well experienced more precompetition cognitive state anxiety than their counterparts who did not perceive such pressure.

Managing Stress In Sports
What Are Signs Of Being Stressed Out?

Sometimes, stress just comes and goes. But if you are facing a lot of pressure or problems, you may start to feel like you're often too stressed out.

Signs that you are getting too stressed may include:

• Feeling down or tired

- Feeling angry or edgy

- Feeling sad or worried

- Having trouble concentrating

- Having headaches or stomach aches

- Having trouble sleeping

- Laughing or crying for no reason

- Wanting to be alone a lot

- Having tense muscles

- Not being able to see the positive side of a situation

- Not enjoying activities that you used to enjoy

- Feeling like you have too many things you have to do

Some of these signs can also be signs of depression, which needs treatment. Learn more about depression and how to get help.

Can Stress Lead To More Serious Problems?

Stress that's too much for you to handle may play a role in some serious problems. These problems include eating disorders, hurting yourself, depression, anxiety disorders, alcohol and drug abuse, smoking, and even suicide. If you are facing any of these problems, talk to an adult you trust right away! You also can get support by phone, text, chat, or email from a special helpline for teens.

How Does My Body Act When Stressed?

Your body has a built-in response to stressors. Your palms may sweat, your mouth may get dry, and your stomach may twist. This is all normal! Of course, stress doesn't feel very good. When your body is hit by stress, try to calm it down. Taking some deep breaths can help. You also can try yoga, going for a walk, or some other physical activity.

Is Stress Always Bad?

- **A little bit of stress can help you.** During a sports competition, stress might push you to perform better, for example. Also, the stress of deadlines can get you to finish work on time.

- **A lot of stress or stress that lasts a long time can hurt you.** It can cause problems for your physical and emotional health, like stomach aches, sleep problems, and trouble concentrating.

- **If your stress is getting to be too much, take steps to tackle it.** Turn to a parent or another adult you trust for advice and support.

- **Don't try to lower your stress in unhealthy ways.** Things like taking drugs, drinking, cutting back on your sleep, or eating a lot or very little will only cause more problems. Treat yourself with the respect you deserve.

Chapter 8

Athletes And Eating Disorders

Eating Disorders

The eating disorders anorexia nervosa, bulimia nervosa, and binge-eating disorder, and their variants, all feature serious disturbances in eating behavior and weight regulation. They are associated with a wide range of adverse psychological, physical, and social consequences. A person with an eating disorder may start out just eating smaller or larger amounts of food, but at some point, their urge to eat less or more spirals out of control. Severe distress or concern about body weight or shape, or extreme efforts to manage weight or food intake, also may characterize an eating disorder.

Eating disorders are real, treatable medical illnesses. They frequently coexist with other illnesses such as depression, substance abuse, or anxiety disorders. Other symptoms can become life-threatening if a person does not receive treatment, which is reflected by anorexia being associated with the highest mortality rate of any psychiatric disorder.

Eating disorders affect both genders, although rates among women and girls are 2½ times greater than among men and boys. Eating disorders frequently appear during the teen years or young adulthood but also may develop during childhood or later in life.

About This Chapter: Text under the heading "Eating Disorders" is excerpted from "Eating Disorders: About More Than Food," National Institute of Mental Health (NIMH), 2014; Texting beginning with the heading "Eating Disorders: A Concern Among Athletes" is excerpted from "Eating Disorders Among Athletes," Education Resources Information Center (ERIC), U.S. Department of Education (ED), June 1, 2013. Reviewed July 2017.

Eat A Healthy Diet

Physical activity, along with a balanced diet, will help you manage your weight. Avoiding excess weight puts less stress on your joints, especially in your knees, hips, and feet. This can help reduce the wear and tear that may lead to arthritis later in life.

Eating a balanced diet will help manage your weight and provide a variety of nutrients for overall health. A balanced diet:

- Emphasizes fruits, vegetables, whole grains, and fat-free or low-fat dairy products like milk, cheese, and yogurt.
- Includes protein from lean meats, poultry, seafood, beans, eggs, and nuts.
- Is low in solid fats, saturated fats, cholesterol, salt (sodium), added sugars, and refined grains.
- Is as low as possible in trans fats.
- Balances calories taken in through food with calories burned in physical activity to help maintain a healthy weight.

(Sources: "Healthy Joints Matter," National Institute of Arthritis and Musculoskeletal and Skin Diseases (NIAMS).)

Eating Disorders: A Concern Among Athletes

Eating disorders among athletes have become a major concern which has evolved due to a number of factors related to athletes and sport performance. First, there is heightened awareness that athletes are human not invincible, and susceptible to a wide variety of problems thought previously to be restricted to the general public. Media coverage has shown that athletes are vulnerable to gambling, alcohol and drug abuses, philandering, and other indulgences perceived as unlawful, immoral, or both. Second, these problems are being exhibited by both professional and amateur athletes at all levels. Third, stellar athletes representing a variety of sports have publicly admitted how devastated they have been by eating disorders or their preoccupation with weight, dieting, and exercise. Many have spoken at college campuses and shared their experiences with others in hopes of bringing attention to the problem and preventing others from replicating their experiences. Fourth, data are beginning to confirm what athletes have been indicating that the problem is not simply isolated to a few individuals hut affects many, both men and women.

In fact, estimates suggest that college athletes are up to six times more likely than the general public to display anorexic or bulimic eating behaviors: men tend to use more aggressive unhealthy approaches to lose weight such as excessive exercise and women rely on more passive means such as fasting, self-induced vomiting, and fad dieting. Fifth, national organizations have expressed their concern about eating disorders and athletes.

Eating Habits Impacts Joints

A joint is where two or more bones are joined together. Joints can be rigid, like the joints between the bones in your skull, or movable, like knees, hips, and shoulders. Many joints have cartilage on the ends of the bones where they come together. Healthy cartilage helps you move by allowing bones to glide over one another. It also protects bones by preventing them from rubbing against each other.

Keeping your joints healthy will allow you to run, walk, jump, play sports, and do the other things you like to do. Physical activity, a balanced diet, avoiding injuries, and getting plenty of sleep will help you stay healthy and keep your joints healthy too.

(Sources: "Healthy Joints Matter," National Institute of Arthritis and Musculoskeletal and Skin Diseases (NIAMS).)

Impact Of Eating Disorders On Athletes

The personal effects of eating disorders may be formally or informally taken into account by athletes. Some athletes may only be partially aware of the consequences of engaging in pathogenic attitudes and behaviors and using unhealthy weight loss methods. Even if athletes engage in a formal decision-making process and calculate the risks, they may believe that the consequences of an eating disorder will not happen to them or if something bad does happen, it will occur in the distant future. Athletes may often focus on the current benefits of their actions (e.g., improved athletic performance) with little regard for future consequences (e.g., personal harm). Consequences of their actions may be ignored in hopes of receiving immediate benefits. The perceived benefits may be even great. For example, athletes may receive recognition, fame, and fortune for maintaining an athletic appearance whether it is worthy or not. These are obviously powerful lures or inducements to counter the impact of ill effects. Unfortunately. the negative as well as the positive consequences occur whether attended to or not. Cumulative research evidence suggests that being eating disordered or engaging in behaviors that mimic an eating disorder can lead to serious physiological and psychological sequelae and even to death.

Chapter 9

The Female Athlete Triad

Being active is great. In fact, girls should be active at least an hour each day. Sometimes, though, a girl will be very active (such as running every day or playing a competitive sport), but not eat enough to fuel her activity. This can lead to health problems. What happens when girls don't eat enough to fuel their activity:

- A problem called "low energy availability"

- Period (menstrual) problems

- Bone problems

These three sometimes are called the female athlete triad. ("Triad" means a group of three). They sometimes also are called Athletic Performance and Energy Deficit. (This means you have a "deficit," or lack, of the energy your body needs to stay healthy.)

A Problem Called "Low Energy Availability"

Your body needs healthy food to fuel the things it does, like fight infections, heal wounds, and grow. If you exercise, your body needs extra food for your workout. You can get learn how much food to eat based on your activity level using the SuperTracker tool (www.choosemyplate.gov/MyPlate-Daily-Checklist).

About This Chapter: Text in this chapter begins with excerpts from "Do You Exercise A Lot?" girlshealth.gov, Office on Women's Health (OWH), March 27, 2015; Text under the heading "Amenorrheic Women And The Female Athlete Triad" is excerpted from "Calcium," Office of Dietary Supplements (ODS), National Institutes of Health (NIH), November 17, 2016.

"Energy availability" means the fuel from food that is not burned up by exercise and so is available for growing, healing, and more. If you exercise a lot and don't get enough nutrition, you may have low energy availability. That means your body won't be as healthy and strong as it should be.

Some female athletes diet to lose weight. They may do this to qualify for their sport or because they think losing weight will help them perform better. But eating enough healthy food is key to having the strength you need to succeed. Also, your body needs good nutrition to make hormones that help with things like healthy periods and strong bones.

Sometimes, girls may exercise too much and eat too little because they have an eating disorder. Eating disorders are serious and can even lead to death, but they are treatable.

Period (Menstrual) Problems

If you are very active, or if you just recently started getting your period (menstruating), you may skip a few periods. But if you work out really hard and do not eat enough, you may skip a lot of periods (or not get your period to begin with) because your body can't make enough of the hormone estrogen.

You may think you wouldn't mind missing your period, but not getting your period should be taken seriously. Not having your period can mean your body is not building enough bone, and the teenage years are the main time for building strong bones.

If you have been getting your period regularly and then miss three periods in a row, see your doctor. Not having your period could be a sign of a serious health problem or of being pregnant. Also see your doctor if you are 15 years old and still have not gotten your period.

Bone Problems

Being physically active helps build strong bones. But you can hurt your bones if you don't eat enough healthy food to fuel all your activity. That's because your body won't be able to make the hormones needed to build strong bones.

One sign that your bones are weak is getting stress fractures, which are tiny cracks in bones. Some places you could get these cracks are your feet, legs, ribs, and spine.

Even if you don't have problems with your bones when you're young, not taking good care of them now can be a problem later in life. Your skeleton is almost completely formed by age 18, so it's important to build strong bones early in life. If you don't, then later on you could wind up with osteoporosis, which is a disease that makes it easier for bones to break.

Signs Of Not Eating Enough And Eating Disorders

Sometimes, girls exercise a lot and do not eat enough because they want to lose weight. Sometimes, exercising just lowers a person's appetite. And sometimes limiting food can be a sign that a girl may be developing an eating disorder. Here are some signs that you or a friend may have a problem:

- Worrying about gaining weight if you don't exercise enough

- Trying harder to find time to exercise than to eat

- Chewing gum or drinking water to cope with hunger

- Often wanting to exercise rather than be with friends

- Exercising instead of doing homework or other responsibilities

- Getting very upset if you miss a workout, but not if you miss a meal

- Having people tell you they are worried you are losing too much weight

If you think you or a friend has a problem, talk to a parent, guardian, or trusted adult.

Sometimes girls exercise a lot because they feel pressure to look a certain way. Soccer star Brandi Chastain knows how bad that can feel. It took a while, she says, for her to realize that only she was in charge of how she felt about her body. "Body image is tough, but it is something we have to take charge of," Brandi says. "Because inside, only we know who we are."

Tips To Prevent Female Athlete Triad

Eat when you're hungry and include a variety of nutrient-rich foods such as lean sources of protein—lean fish, poultry, beans, nuts, and low-fat dairy products—along with whole grains, fruits, and vegetables. Skipping meals and snacks or severely restricting your food intake will keep you from getting enough calories and other important nutrients such as protein, vitamins, and minerals.

Eat a recovery snack that consists of carbs and protein after your workout. Carbs are your body's primary fuel source to keep you energized, and you need protein to build and repair your muscles.

Talk to a registered dietitian for an individual nutrition plan. A registered dietitian who specializes in sports nutrition can help you choose the best foods and the right amounts to optimize your performance.

(Source: "Are You At Risk For Female Athlete Triad?" Military Health System (MHS).)

Amenorrheic Women And The Female Athlete Triad

Amenorrhea, the condition in which menstrual periods stop or fail to initiate in women of childbearing age, results from reduced circulating estrogen levels that, in turn, have a negative effect on calcium balance. Amenorrheic women with anorexia nervosa have decreased calcium absorption and higher urinary calcium excretion rates, as well as a lower rate of bone formation than healthy women. The "female athlete triad" refers to the combination of disordered eating, amenorrhea, and osteoporosis. Exercise-induced amenorrhea generally results in decreased bone mass. In female athletes and active women in the military, low bone-mineral density, menstrual irregularities, certain dietary patterns, and a history of prior stress fractures are associated with an increased risk of future stress fractures. Such women should be advised to consume adequate amounts of calcium and vitamin D. Supplements of these nutrients have been shown to reduce the risk of stress fractures in female Navy recruits during basic training.

Chapter 10

Abuse In Sports

What Is Abuse?

The Child Abuse Prevention and Treatment Act (CAPTA) defines child abuse and neglect as, "any recent act or failure to act on the part of a parent or caretaker which results in death, serious physical or emotional harm, sexual abuse or exploitation" or "an act or failure to act which presents an imminent risk of serious harm." Any kind of physical, emotional, sexual maltreatment, neglect, or harassment that leads to harm is considered abuse. Abuse takes place in many startling ways in the world of youth sports.

What Is Emotional Abuse?

Any behavior that damages the sense of self-worth of a child is considered emotional abuse. Emotional abuse is the most common form of injury affecting youth in sports. It occurs when a parent, sibling, caregiver, guardian, or coach behaves negatively with a child. Some forms of emotional abuse are listed below.

- Forcing an otherwise unwilling child to participate in sports
- Yelling at a child for not performing well or losing
- Meting out punishment for mediocre performance or losing a game
- Ridiculing or criticizing moves on the field
- Ignoring, rejecting, or isolating a child
- Withholding love, support, and guidance

"Abuse In Sports," © 2017 Omnigraphics. Reviewed July 2017.

- Engaging in name-calling

- Being taunted or bullied by teammates

- Insulting a child for not meeting expectations

- Being intimidated by teammates or their guardians

- Hazing

Emotional abuse affects the development of children and triggers negative emotions such as anger, anxiety, guilt, sadness, shame, envy, jealousy, fright, and disgust. Such children are emotionally vulnerable and are at a greater risk of developing psychiatric illnesses later in life.

What Is Physical Abuse?

Physical abuse happens when someone deliberately injures a child by hitting, shaking, throwing, biting, burning, scalding, suffocating, or drowning him or her. Sports training so intense that it cannot be borne by the body is considered physical abuse. Coaches who promote performance-enhancing drugs are also essentially engaging in physical abuse. Forcing athletes to participate in events despite injury and imposing sanctions that inflict pain for nonperformance are considered physical abuse as well.

Sexual Abuse In Sports

In sports and other youth activities, children and teens could be sexually abused by adults or peers. Sexual abusers in this setting often use their position of authority or trust to first gain the confidence of the victim and that of their parents or caregivers. Then they use this same authority to keep the child from reporting the abuse.

In youth sports, coaches will invariably come into close physical contact with students. Responsible coaches respect the privacy of their athletes and keep their physical interactions with their team minimal and nurturing. Abusers, on the other hand, will take advantage of the closeness to act, often without being discovered (e.g., kissing or fondling a student as a form of "praise," abusing students while traveling for a game or secretly filming students changing in locker rooms, etc.).

What Is Harassment?

Harassment of children involves threats, taunts, intimidation, and usage of homophobic, sexist, and racial slurs by others. Comments, behavior, and contact that are uninvited, unwelcome, offensive, and sexual in nature also constitute harassment.

What Is Neglect?

Neglect occurs when caretakers, parents, or guardians fail to meet the basic physical and psychological needs of children. In youth sports, children are neglected when supervisors or coaches fail to follow basic safety guidelines and use protective equipment. Forcing children to play and practice in adverse weather conditions without sufficient protection or hydration is also neglect. Requiring children to play in spite of being unwell or ignoring bullying by teammates can be considered neglect.

Coaches and administrators must also act responsibly to minimize risk for students. Injuries such as concussions are a case in point. It would be better to have the player taken off the ground and sent for medical diagnosis than to convince him or her to "shake it off" and continue playing.

What Is Philosophical Abuse In Sports?

Following the rules of the game, treating everyone (teammates, coaches, opponents, referees, and fans) with respect, and giving your all on the field are the founding principles of sportsmanship. Most coaches and parents make sure children understand that sportsmanship always outweighs winning at all costs. However, when adults repeatedly want to know if they won, what was the score, and punish or belittle the youth if they do not win, children acquire the false notion that self-worth is built only upon winning. The spirit of sportsmanship can be greatly beneficial to the psychological health of children and is worth making it a centerpiece of any sports program.

What Is The Kind Of Misconduct Seen In Sports Events?

Parents who verbally abuse or physically confront students and coaches at sporting events are becoming an increasingly common. Surveys conducted recently indicate that a significant percentage of coaches have experienced parents behaving inappropriately, including yelling at or taunting children on the field, confronting referees, or physically attacking coaches or other parents.

For children of parents who act in the manner, regularly witnessing, or being the target, this behavior increases the chances of being diagnosed with anxiety or depression. It also increases the likelihood of them engaging in risky behaviors such as aggression and delinquency.

How Can Abuse In Youth Sports Be Prevented?

It is up to parents, coaches, and educators to teach children about what constitutes acceptable behavior and to protect them for abuse and exploitation. It is the responsibility of parents as well to understand the attitude of coaches and others who train and supervise their children.

Organizations, such as schools and sports leagues, must also recognize the fact that children can be vulnerable to abuse and it should make it a priority to put into place preventative programs. The Centers for Disease Control and Prevention (CDC) has defined six key components for the creation of an environment and culture in youth-focused organizations that can contribute to the prevention of child abuse. These include the following.

1. Screening and selecting employees and volunteers for past convictions for abuse.

2. Setting guidelines on interactions between adults and youth and what constitutes appropriate behavior among youth themselves.

3. Monitoring behavior to respond to risky behaviors and reinforce positive ones.

4. Ensuring safe environments to protect children from situations that can be high risk for abuse.

5. Responding quickly and responsibly to inappropriate behavior, breaches in policy, and allegations or suspicion of child sexual abuse.

6. Training staff and stakeholders about child sexual abuse prevention so they can respond responsibly to issues of child abuse.

Programs should be assessed and reviewed periodically for effectiveness.

References

1. "Emotional Abuse in Youth Sports," Focus Adolescent Services, n.d.

2. de Lench, Brooke. "Abuse in Youth Sports Takes Many Different Forms," MomsTEAM Institute, Inc., n.d.

3. "Child Abuse in a Sports Setting," National Society for the Prevention of Cruelty to Children (NSPCC), 2017.

4. Aron, Cindy Miller. "Mind, Body and Sport: The Haunting Legacy of Abuse," The National Collegiate Athletic Association (NCAA), n.d.

5. "Definitions of Child Abuse and Neglect in Federal Law," Child Welfare Information Gateway, n.d.

6. "Preventing Child Abuse in Youth Sports," SI Play, LLC., 2017.

7. "Kidpower Teams Up with Positive Coaching Alliance (PCA) To Stop Child Abuse in Youth Sports," Kidpower Teenpower Fullpower International, June 5, 2012.

8. "Preventing Child Sexual Abuse Within Youth-serving Organizations: Getting Started on Policies and Procedures," Centers for Disease Control and Prevention, 2007.

Chapter 11

Overtraining Syndrome (Athlete Burnout)

Overtraining Syndrome[1]

Are you the type of athlete that has a need to always practice, weight lift, or do some kind of cardiovascular workout? Does your mind tell you that training and training and more training will make you feel better? Do you also tell yourself that rest or sitting around is bad for you? If you answered yes, you might have what is known as overtraining syndrome, "staleness," or "burnout."

Risk Factors[1]

Overtraining occurs when there is a continuous, excessive overload of exercise without proper rest and proper nutrition. Many people fail to adapt to the stress sustained during high intensity training because they don't give their bodies enough time to adapt and recuperate. A poorly designed program consisting of a rapid increase in volume and intensity, consistently high volume training, and insufficient time for rest and recovery can lead to the body shutting down. Other factors that will increase your chances for developing overtraining syndrome are frequent competition, preexisting medical conditions, poor diet, environmental stress, and psychosocial stress.

About This Chapter: This chapter includes text excerpted from documents published by two public domain sources. Text under headings marked 1 are excerpted from "Feeling 'Stale' From Overtraining," National Aeronautics and Space Administration (NASA), n.d. Reviewed July 2017; Text under heading marked 2 is excerpted from "Exercise And Bone Health For Women: The Skeletal Risk Of Overtraining," National Institute of Arthritis and Musculoskeletal and Skin Diseases (NIAMS), May 2016.

The Skeletal Risk Of Overtraining In Female Athletes[2]

Girls and women who engage in rigorous exercise regimens or who try to lose weight by restricting their eating are at risk for these health problems. They may include serious athletes, "gym rats" (who spend considerable time and energy working out), and girls and women who believe "you can never be too thin."

Some athletes see amenorrhea (the absence of menstrual periods) as a sign of successful training. Others see it as a great answer to a monthly inconvenience. And some young women accept it blindly, not stopping to think of the consequences. But missing your periods is often a sign of decreased estrogen levels. And lower estrogen levels can lead to osteoporosis, a disease in which your bones become brittle and more likely to break.

Usually, bones don't become brittle and break until women are much older. But some young women, especially those who exercise so much that their periods stop, develop brittle bones, and may start to have fractures at a very early age. Some 20-year-old female athletes have been said to have the bones of an 80-year-old woman. Even if bones don't break when you're young, low estrogen levels during the peak years of bone-building, the preteen and teen years, can affect bone density for the rest of your life. And studies show that bone growth lost during these years may never be regained.

Broken bones don't just hurt—they can cause lasting physical malformations. Have you noticed that some older women and men have stooped postures? This is not a normal sign of aging. Fractures from osteoporosis have left their spines permanently altered.

Signs Of Burnout[1]

With all these factors and living in a world filled with stress, how do you know if you have this syndrome? There are many signs and symptoms with overtraining, but the primary element is the unpredicted drop in performance. A person can train and compete at the same level as they are use to, but they will have greater difficulty in maintaining the performance. Other signs and symptoms include excessive muscle fatigue, increased resting heart rate, trouble sleeping, depression, anxiety, increased weight loss, frequent injuries, and illnesses.

Treatment[1]

Overtraining syndrome is not something that is hard to treat. First off, it is always wise to consult a physician if it is suspected. This can rule out any disease or illness that can be caused by overtraining. Recovery will take at least two weeks depending on how severe the case is. Your activities should be extremely limited, if not discontinued during this time frame, and proper rest and nutrition should be given. A diet of low fat and high carbohydrates is recommended because of the depleted glycogen level over the period of time.

Prevention[1]

Early recognition will prevent any damages that could affect the body. To prevent overtraining from occurring, have an alternative workout schedule with proper rest for the body in between. Training should alternate from a heavy workday to a light workday. Good nutrition complete with complex carbohydrates, fruits, vegetables, and protein should be part of the diet. Proper hydration is a must! A person exercising should take in at least 8 servings, 12 fl oz. each, of water per pound lost. Increases in training should be progressed slowly so the body has time to adapt. To increase in training, one should use the 10 percent rule. The 10 percent rule is an increase of 10 percent in either intensity, duration or volume in one workout session at a time. Intensity, duration, and volume should not be increased at the same time. Most importantly, educating yourself about proper exercise is a key. And listen to your body... It will tell you when it's had enough!

Chapter 12

Anabolic Steroids

What Are Anabolic Steroids?

Anabolic steroids are synthetic variations of the male sex hormone testosterone. The proper term for these compounds is *anabolic-androgenic steroids*. "Anabolic" refers to muscle building, and "androgenic" refers to increased male sex characteristics. Some common names for anabolic steroids are Gear, Juice, Roids, and Stackers.

Healthcare providers can prescribe steroids to treat hormonal issues, such as delayed puberty. Steroids can also treat diseases that cause muscle loss, such as cancer and acquired immune deficiency syndrome (AIDS). But some athletes and bodybuilders abuse these drugs to boost performance or improve their physical appearance.

How Do People Abuse Anabolic Steroids?

People who abuse anabolic steroids usually take them orally or inject them into the muscles. These doses may be 10 to 100 times higher than doses prescribed to treat medical conditions. Steroids are also applied to the skin as a cream, gel, or patch.

Some athletes and others who abuse steroids believe that they can avoid unwanted side effects or maximize the drugs' effects by taking them in ways that include:

- cycling—taking doses for a period of time, stopping for a time, and then restarting

- stacking—combining two or more different types of steroids

About This Chapter: This chapter includes text excerpted from "Anabolic Steroids," National Institute on Drug Abuse (NIDA), March 2016.

- pyramiding—slowly increasing the dose or frequency of abuse, reaching a peak amount, and then gradually tapering off

There is no scientific evidence that any of these practices reduce the harmful medical consequences of these drugs.

How Do Anabolic Steroids Affect The Brain?

Anabolic steroids work differently from other drugs of abuse; they do not have the same short-term effects on the brain. The most important difference is that steroids do not trigger rapid increases in the brain chemical dopamine, which causes the "high" that drives people to abuse other substances. However, long-term steroid abuse can act on some of the same brain pathways and chemicals—including dopamine, serotonin, and opioid systems—that are affected by other drugs. This may result in a significant effect on mood and behavior.

Short-Term Effects

Abuse of anabolic steroids may lead to mental problems, such as:

- paranoid (extreme, unreasonable) jealousy
- extreme irritability
- delusions—false beliefs or ideas
- impaired judgment

Extreme mood swings can also occur, including "roid rage"—angry feelings and behavior that may lead to violence.

What Are The Other Health Effects Of Anabolic Steroids?

Aside from mental problems, steroid use commonly causes severe acne. It also causes the body to swell, especially in the hands and feet.

Long-Term Effects

Anabolic steroid abuse may lead to serious, even permanent, health problems such as:

- kidney problems or failure
- liver damage

- enlarged heart, high blood pressure, and changes in blood cholesterol, all of which increase the risk of stroke and heart attack, even in young people

Several other effects are gender- and age-specific:

- In teens:
  - stunted growth (when high hormone levels from steroids signal to the body to stop bone growth too early)
  - stunted height (if teens use steroids before their growth spurt)

Some of these physical changes, such as shrinking sex organs in men, can add to mental side effects such as mood disorders.

Anabolic Steroids And Infectious Diseases

People who inject steroids increase their risk of contracting or transmitting human immuno-deficiency virus (HIV)/AIDS or hepatitis.

Are Anabolic Steroids Addictive?

Even though anabolic steroids do not cause the same high as other drugs, they can lead to addiction. Studies have shown that animals will self-administer steroids when they have the chance, just as they do with other addictive drugs. People may continue to abuse steroids despite physical problems, high costs to buy the drugs, and negative effects on their relationships. These behaviors reflect steroids' addictive potential. Research has further found that some steroid users turn to other drugs, such as opioids, to reduce sleep problems and irritability caused by steroids.

People who abuse steroids may experience withdrawal symptoms when they stop use, including:

- mood swings
- fatigue
- restlessness
- loss of appetite
- sleep problems

- decreased sex drive

- steroid cravings

One of the more serious withdrawal symptoms is depression, which can sometimes lead to suicide attempts.

How Can People Get Treatment For Anabolic Steroid Addiction?

Some people seeking treatment for anabolic steroid addiction have found behavioral therapy to be helpful. More research is needed to identify the most effective treatment options.

In certain cases of severe addiction, patients have taken medicines to help treat symptoms of withdrawal. For example, healthcare providers have prescribed antidepressants to treat depression and pain medicines for headaches and muscle and joint pain. Other medicines have been used to help restore the patient's hormonal system.

Chapter 13

Alcohol And Marijuana: Problems For Teen Athletes

Underage Drinking

Alcohol is by far the drug of choice among youth. It's often the first one tried, and it's used by the most kids. Over the course of adolescence, the proportion of kids who drank in the previous year rises tenfold, from 7 percent of 12-year-olds to nearly 70 percent of 18-year-olds. Dangerous binge drinking is common and increases with age as well: About 1 in 14 eighth graders, 1 in 6 tenth graders, and 1 in 4 twelfth graders report having five or more drinks in a row in the past 2 weeks.

> Youth engage in binge drinking, a pattern of drinking that elevates the blood alcohol concentration to 0.08 percent or above, more than adults do. This can lead to risky and potentially harmful behaviors, and many times substance abuse (60–75 percent of youth with substance abuse problems) cooccurs with mental health disorders.
>
> *(Source: "Substance Abuse Prevention," Youth.gov.)*

It's Risky

In the short term, adolescent drinking too often results in unintentional injuries and death; suicidality; aggression and victimization; infections and pregnancies from unplanned,

About This Chapter: Text under the heading "Underage Drinking" is excerpted from "Alcohol Screening And Brief Intervention For Youth—A Practitioner's Guide," National Institute on Alcohol Abuse and Alcoholism (NIAAA), October 2015; Text under the heading "Athletes And Alcohol And Other Drug Usage" is excerpted from "College Athletes And Alcohol And Other Drug Use," Education Resources Information Center (ERIC), U.S. Department of Education (ED), August 2008. Reviewed July 2017; Text under the heading "Being A Team Player Can Influence Drug And Alcohol Use" is excerpted from "Drugs & Health Blog—Being a Team Player Can Influence Drug and Alcohol Use," National Institute on Drug Abuse (NIDA) for Teens, June 20, 2012. Reviewed July 2017.

unprotected sex; and academic and social problems. In the long term, drinking in adolescence is associated with increased risk for alcohol dependence later in life. In addition, heavy drinking in adolescence may result in long-lasting functional and structural changes in the brain.

Athletes And Alcohol And Other Drug Usage

Few would argue that athletic success depends on both physical and mental health. Given that, it would be reasonable to expect that college athletes avoid using alcohol and other drugs to preserve their overall health and enhance their athletic performance. In fact, college athletes use alcohol, spit tobacco, and steroids at higher rates than their non-athlete peers. Cocaine attracted publicity for its role in the deaths of star athletes in the 1980s and has since waned as a prevalent drug among college athletes. Even so, cocaine still poses risks for college athletes, as do other drugs such as diet aids, ephedrine, marijuana, and psychedelics.

Alcohol

A national study of varsity athletes found that almost 77 percent of athletes had used alcohol in the previous 12 months, a decrease from 81 percent. A national study of college student drinking found that athletes have significantly higher rates of heavy drinking (defined as five or more drinks in a row for men, four or more for women) than non-athletes. Among men not competing in intercollegiate athletics, 49 percent reported heavy drinking in the two weeks prior to the survey, compared with 57 percent of the male athletes. For women students, the difference in drinking patterns was just as disparate: 40 percent of non-athlete women reported heavy drinking in the previous two weeks, compared with 48 percent of female athletes. Athletes tend to drink in seasonal cycles. A study at a large private university found an approximate 50 percent increase in drinking when athletes were off-season. In season, 42 percent of men and 26 percent of women drank alcohol at least once a week, but during the remainder of the year weekly alcohol consumption jumped to 60 percent for men and 41 percent for women.

Spit Tobacco

Although spit tobacco is often marketed as "smokeless tobacco," implying that it poses fewer health risks than cigarettes, chewing tobacco and snuff are highly addictive and can lead to oral cancer, mouth lesions, and gum disease. Male athletes are particularly at risk, chiefly because of intensive marketing targeted to adolescent boys, distribution of free spit tobacco to college players, promotions by professional athletes, and the convenience of using spit tobacco during games. A national study found spit tobacco to be widely used among male college athletes, especially baseball players. Fully 42 percent of baseball players and 30 percent of football players had used spit tobacco in the previous 12 months. These figures are a drop from nearly 60 percent of baseball players and 40 percent of football players in the early 1990s, yet they still dwarf the national use rate of 17 percent for college men. In most women's sports, spit tobacco use is rare, but in the same national study, nearly 20 percent of women ice hockey players reported using. A survey of varsity baseball players at 52 California colleges found clear racial and ethnic differences in spit tobacco use: 42 percent of white athletes, 37 percent of Asians, 36 percent of Hispanics, 35 percent of Native American and 11 percent of African Americans use spit tobacco. Almost 98 percent of the athletes who use spit tobacco started by the age of 20.

Anabolic Steroids And Amphetamines

An National Collegiate Athletic Association (NCAA) national study found that anabolic steroids are not widely used by intercollegiate athletes. The user rate was 1 percent, a significant drop from 5 percent. Still, this rate is more than triple the national rate by non-athlete students. Two percent of male football players used anabolic steroids, a drop from nearly 10 percent. Athletes maintained the same usage rate of amphetamines, hovering at 3 percent, between 1989 and 2001. The rate increased to 4 percent in 2005. The sport with the most amphetamine use by men is rifle shooting, with 8 percent of participants using. Among female athletes, the most prevalent use was by softball players, at about 5 percent.

Marijuana

Past NCAA surveys revealed a sharp decrease in marijuana use between the late 1980s and early 1990s. In a reversal of that trend, more than 28 percent of the athletes surveyed in 1997 reported using marijuana at least once during the previous year. This figure dropped to 20 percent in 2005. The majority of the athletes surveyed in 2005 had started using marijuana prior to coming to college. Specifically, 66 percent of users started in high school, 12 percent started during their freshman year in college, and 6 percent after their freshman year in college. By ethnic group, the highest rate of marijuana use was found among Caucasians. Among athletes, 63 percent of marijuana users said they use the drug to serve recreational or social purposes and 35 percent said that they use it because it makes them feel good. Among those not using marijuana, 15 percent said they refrained because they had no desire for the drug's effects, 37 percent refrained because they were concerned about their health, and 11 percent refrained because it was against their religious or moral beliefs.

Being A Team Player Can Influence Drug And Alcohol Use

Middle and high school teens have many choices when it comes to extracurricular activities. Some will choose a team sport like basketball, volleyball, football, or softball, while others may choose more individual-type sports like track, golf, tennis, or swimming.

Either way, being an athlete can be a positive experience—it teaches the importance of cooperation and practice, and how to win and lose gracefully—and it helps keep your body healthy. A study reports it may also influence decisions about using drugs like cigarettes, marijuana, or alcohol—but the news is not all good.

The good news is that researchers found that students who participate in team sports or exercise regularly report much less cigarette smoking than students not involved in sports. Also, fewer student athletes used marijuana.

The bad news is that the same study showed the reverse when it comes to drinking alcohol—that student athletes were much more likely to drink alcohol than non-athletes. This may be because team sports often involve alcohol—while watching the event or celebrating afterwards. That's why beer companies are major sponsors of pro sports teams.

Drugs And Alcohol Can Slow You Down

By now, most of us know that smoking cigarettes affects athletes' abilities in several ways, causing problems with breathing and endurance, for example. And marijuana can compromise your balance, perception, and memory, making it hard to be physically or mentally at your best in competition.

However, as the study points out, some high school athletes don't realize that drinking alcohol also impairs both physical and mental conditioning.

Your body and brain may not respond the way you need them to after you use drugs or drink alcohol.

Chapter 14

Teen Athletes And The Use Of Dietary Supplements

This chapter provides an overview of selected ingredients in dietary supplements designed or claimed to enhance exercise and athletic performance. Manufacturers and sellers promote these products, sometimes referred to as "ergogenic aids," by claiming that they improve strength or endurance, increase exercise efficiency, achieve a performance goal more quickly, and increase tolerance for more intense training. These effects are the main focus of this fact sheet. Some people also use ergogenic aids to prepare the body for exercise, reduce the chance of injury during training, and enhance recovery from exercise.

Dietary supplements to enhance exercise and athletic performance come in a variety of forms, including tablets, capsules, liquids, powders, and bars. Many of these products contain numerous ingredients in varied combinations and amounts. Among the more common ingredients are amino acids, protein, creatine, and caffeine. According to one estimate, retail sales of the category of "sports nutrition supplements" totaled $5.67 billion in 2016, or 13.8 percent of $41.16 billion total sales for dietary supplements and related nutrition products for that year.

Several surveys have indicated the extent of dietary supplement use for bodybuilding and to enhance exercise and athletic performance:

- International surveys found that two-thirds of 3,887 adult and adolescent elite track and field athletes participating in world-championship competitions took one or more dietary supplements containing such ingredients as vitamins, minerals, creatine, caffeine, and amino acids. Supplement use increased with age and was significantly more common among women than men.

About This Chapter: This chapter includes text excerpted from "Dietary Supplements For Exercise And Athletic Performance," Office of Dietary Supplements (ODS), National Institutes of Health (NIH), June 30, 2017.

- A survey of 1,248 students aged 16 years or older in five U.S. colleges and universities in 2009–2010 found that 66 percent reported use of any dietary supplement. The reasons for use included enhanced muscle strength (20% of users), performance enhancement (19% of users), and increased endurance (7% of users). Products taken for these purposes included protein, amino acids, herbal supplements, caffeine, creatine, and combination products.

- In a national survey of about 21,000 U.S. college athletes, respondents reported taking protein products (41.7%), energy drinks and shots (28.6%), creatine (14.0%), amino acids (12.1%), multivitamins with caffeine (5.7%), beta-hydroxy-beta-methylbutyrate (HMB; 0.2%), dehydroepiandrosterone (DHEA; 0.1%), and an unspecified mix of "testosterone boosters" (1.6%). Men were much more likely to take performance-enhancing products than women, except for energy drinks and shots. Among the sports with the highest percentage of users of performance-enhancing products were ice hockey, wrestling, and baseball among the men and volleyball, swimming, and ice hockey among the women.

- In a review of studies on adolescent use of performance-enhancing substances, the American Academy of Pediatrics concluded that protein, creatine, and caffeine were the most commonly used ingredients and that use increased with age. Although athletes used these ingredients more than nonathletes, teenagers not involved in organized athletic activities often took them to enhance their appearance.

- A survey of 106,698 U.S. military personnel in 2007–2008 found that 22.8 percent of the men and 5.3 percent of the women reported using bodybuilding supplements, such as creatine and amino acids, and 40.5 percent of the men and 35.5 percent of the women reported using energy supplements that might contain caffeine and/or energy-enhancing herbs. Use of these products was positively associated with deployment to combat situations, being younger than 29 years, being physically active, and reporting 5 or fewer hours of sleep a night.

It is difficult to make generalizations about the extent of dietary supplement use by athletes because the studies on this topic are heterogeneous. But the data suggest that:

- A larger proportion of athletes than the general U.S. population takes dietary supplements.

- Elite athletes (e.g., professional athletes and those who compete on a national or international level) use dietary supplements more often than their nonelite counterparts.

- The supplements used by male and female athletes are similar, except that a larger proportion of women use iron and a larger proportion of men take vitamin E, protein, and creatine.

For any individual to physically perform at his or her best, a nutritionally adequate diet and sufficient hydration are critical. The *Dietary Guidelines for Americans* and MyPlate recommend such an eating plan for everyone. Athletes require adequate daily amounts of calories, fluids, carbohydrates (to maintain blood glucose levels and replace muscle glycogen; typically 1.4 to 4.5 g/lb body weight [3 to 10 g/kg body weight]), protein (0.55 to 0.9 g/lb body weight [1.2 to 2.0 g/kg body weight]), fat (20% to 35% of total calories), and vitamins and minerals.

A few dietary supplements might enhance performance only when they add to, but do not substitute for, this dietary foundation. Athletes engaging in endurance activities lasting more than an hour or performed in extreme environments (e.g., hot temperatures or high altitudes) might need to replace lost fluids and electrolytes and consume additional carbohydrates for energy. Even with proper nutritional preparation, the results of taking any dietary supplement(s) for exercise and athletic performance vary by level of training; the nature, intensity, and duration of the activity; and the environmental conditions.

Sellers claim that dozens of ingredients in dietary supplements can enhance exercise and athletic performance. Well-trained elite and recreational athletes might use products containing one or more of these ingredients to train harder, improve performance, and achieve a competitive edge. However, the National Athletic Trainers' Association acknowledges in a position statement that because the outcomes of studies of various performance-enhancing substances are often equivocal, using these substances can be "controversial and confusing."

Most studies to assess the potential value and safety of supplements to enhance exercise and athletic performance include only conditioned athletes. Therefore, it is often not clear whether the supplements discussed in this chapter may be of value to recreational exercisers or individuals who engage in athletic activity only occasionally. In addition, much of the research on these supplements involves young adults (more often male than female), and not adolescents who may also use them against the advice of pediatric and high-school professional associations. The quality of many studies is limited by their small samples and short durations, use of performance tests that do not simulate real-world conditions or are unreliable or irrelevant, and poor control of confounding variables. Furthermore, the benefits and risks shown for the supplements might not apply to the supplement's use to enhance types of physical performance not assessed in the studies. In most cases, additional research is needed to fully understand the efficacy and safety of particular ingredients.

Selected Ingredients In Dietary Supplements For Exercise And Athletic Performance

Many exercise and athletic-performance dietary supplements in the marketplace contain multiple ingredients (especially those marketed for muscle growth and strength). However, much of the research has focused only on single ingredients. One therefore cannot know or predict the effects and safety of combinations in these multi-ingredient products unless clinical trials have investigated that particular combination. Furthermore, the amounts of these ingredients vary widely among products. In some cases, the products contain proprietary blends of ingredients listed in order by weight, but labels do not provide the amount of each ingredient in the blend. Manufacturers and sellers of dietary supplements for exercise and athletic performance rarely fund or conduct scientific research on their proprietary products of a caliber that reputable biomedical journals require for publication.

Table 14.1 briefly summarizes the findings discussed in more detail in this fact sheet on the safety and efficacy of selected ingredients in dietary supplements to enhance exercise and athletic performance. Some research-derived data is available on these ingredients on which to base a judgment about their potential value to aid exercise and athletic performance. These dietary supplement ingredients are listed and discussed in the table, and in the text that follows the table, in alphabetical order.

Table 14.1. Selected Ingredients In Dietary Supplements For Exercise And Athletic Performance

Ingredient	Proposed Mechanism Of Action	Evidence Of Efficacy*	Evidence Of Safety*
Antioxidants (vitamin C, vitamin E, and coenzyme Q10)	Minimize free-radical damage to skeletal muscle, thereby reducing muscle fatigue, inflammation, and soreness	Several small clinical trials Research findings: Do not directly improve performance; appear to hinder some physiological and physical exercise-induced adaptations	Safe at recommended intakes; some safety concerns reported with high doses Reported adverse effects: Potential for diarrhea, nausea, abdominal cramps, and other gastrointestinal disturbances with vitamin C intakes of more than 2,000 mg/day in adults; increased risk of hemorrhagic effects with vitamin E intakes of more than 1,500 IU/day (natural form) or 1,100 IU/day (synthetic form) in adults; nausea, heartburn, and other side effects with coenzyme Q10
Arginine	Increases blood flow and delivery of oxygen and nutrients to skeletal muscle; serves as a substrate for creatine production; increases secretion of human growth hormone to stimulate muscle growth	Limited clinical trials with conflicting results Research findings: Little to no effect on vasodilation, blood flow, or exercise metabolites; little evidence of increases in muscle creatine content	No safety concerns reported for use of up to 9 g/day for weeks; adverse effects possible with larger doses Reported adverse effects: Gastrointestinal effects, such as diarrhea and nausea

Table 14.1. Continued

Ingredient	Proposed Mechanism Of Action	Evidence Of Efficacy*	Evidence Of Safety*
Beetroot or beet juice	Dilates blood vessels in exercising muscle, reduces oxygen use, and improves energy production	Limited clinical trials with conflicting results Research findings: Might improve performance and endurance to some degree in time trials and time-to-exhaustion tests among runners, swimmers, rowers, and cyclists; appears to be most effective in recreationally active non-athletes	No safety concerns reported for short-term use at commonly recommended amounts (approximately 2 cups) Reported adverse effects: None known
Beta-alanine	Increases synthesis of carnosine, a dipeptide that buffers changes in muscle pH, thereby reducing muscle fatigue and loss of force production; considerable individual variation in associated muscle carnosine synthesis	Numerous clinical trials with conflicting results Research findings: Inconsistent effects on performance in competitive events requiring high-intensity effort over a short period, such as team sports; little or no performance benefit in activities lasting more than 10 minutes	No safety concerns reported for use of 1.6–6.4 g/day for up to 8 weeks Reported adverse effects: Paresthesia (tingling) in face, neck, back of hands, and upper trunk with at least 800 mg or over 10 mg/kg body mass; pruritus (itchy skin)
Beta-hydroxy-beta(HMB)-methylbutyrate	Helps stressed and damaged skeletal muscle cells restore their structure and function	Numerous clinical trials with conflicting results Research findings: Might help speed up recovery from exercise of sufficient amount and intensity to induce skeletal muscle damage	No safety concerns reported for typical dose of 3 g/day for up to 2 months Reported adverse effects: None known

Table 14.1. Continued

Ingredient	Proposed Mechanism Of Action	Evidence Of Efficacy*	Evidence Of Safety*
Betaine	Might increase creatine production, blood nitric-acid levels, or water retention in cells	Limited clinical trials in men with conflicting results Research findings: Potential but modest strength and power-based performance improvements in bodybuilders and cyclists	No safety concerns reported for 2–5 g/day for up to 15 days Reported adverse effects: None known
Branched-chain amino acids (leucine, isoleucine, and valine)	Can be metabolized by mitochondria in skeletal muscle to provide energy during exercise	Limited number of short-term clinical trials Research findings: Little evidence of improved performance in endurance-related aerobic events; possibility of greater gains in muscle mass and strength during training	No safety concerns reported for 20 g/day or less for up to 6 weeks Reported adverse effects: None known
Caffeine	Blocks activity of the neuromodulator adenosine; reduces perceived pain and exertion	Numerous clinical trials with mostly consistent results Research findings: Might enhance performance in endurance-type activities (e.g., running) and intermittent, long-duration activities (e.g., soccer) when taken before activity	Reasonably safe at up to 400–500 mg/day for adults Reported adverse effects: Insomnia, restlessness, nausea, vomiting, tachycardia, and arrhythmia; risk of death with acute oral dose of approximately 10–14 g pure caffeine (150–200 mg/kg)

Table 14.1. Continued

Ingredient	Proposed Mechanism Of Action	Evidence Of Efficacy*	Evidence Of Safety*
Citrulline	Dilates blood vessels to increase delivery of oxygen and nutrients to skeletal muscle	Few clinical trials with conflicting results Research findings: Little research support for use to enhance performance	Few safety concerns reported for up to 9 g for 1 day or 6 g/day for up to 16 days Reported adverse effects: Gastrointestinal discomfort
Creatine	Helps supply muscles with energy for short-term, predominantly anaerobic activity	Numerous clinical trials generally showing a benefit for high-intensity, intermittent activity; potential variation in individual responses Research findings: May increase strength, power, and work from maximal effort muscle contractions; over time helps body adapt to athlete-training regimens; of little value for endurance sports	Few safety concerns reported at typical dose (e.g., loading dose of 20 g/day for up to 7 days and 3–5 g/day for up to 12 weeks) Reported adverse effects: Weight gain due to water retention; anecdotal reports of nausea, diarrhea, muscle cramps, muscle stiffness, heat intolerance
Deer antler velvet	Contains growth factors (such as insulin-like growth factor-1 [IGF-1]) that could promote muscle tissue growth	Few short-term clinical trials that show no benefit for physical performance Research findings: No evidence for improving aerobic or anaerobic performance, muscular strength, or endurance	Safety not well studied Reported adverse effects: Hypoglycemia, headache, edema, and joint pain (from prescription IGF-1); banned in professional athletic competition

Table 14.1. Continued

Ingredient	Proposed Mechanism Of Action	Evidence Of Efficacy*	Evidence Of Safety*
Dehydroepiandrosterone (DHEA)	Steroid hormone that can be converted into testosterone and estradiol	Small number of clinical trials that show no benefit for physical performance Research findings: No evidence of increases in strength, aerobic capacity, lean body mass, or testosterone levels in men	Safety not well studied; no safety concerns reported for up to 150 mg/day for 6–12 weeks Reported adverse effects: Over several months, raises testosterone levels in women, which can cause acne and growth of facial hair
Ginseng	Unknown mechanism of action; Panax ginseng used in traditional Chinese medicine as a tonic for stamina and vitality; Siberian ginseng used to reduce fatigue	Numerous small clinical trials, most showing no benefit for physical performance Research findings: In various doses and types of preparations, no effects on peak power output, time to exhaustion, perceived exertion, recovery from intense activity, oxygen consumption, or heart rate	Few safety concerns reported with short-term use Reported adverse effects: For Panax ginseng: headache, sleep disturbances, and gastrointestinal disorders; for Siberian ginseng: none known

Table 14.1. Continued

Ingredient	Proposed Mechanism Of Action	Evidence Of Efficacy*	Evidence Of Safety*
Glutamine	Involved in metabolism and energy production; contributes nitrogen for many critical biochemical reactions	Few studies of use to enhance performance directly Research findings: In adult weight lifters, no effect on muscle performance, body composition, or muscle-protein degradation; may help with recovery of muscle strength and reduce muscle soreness after exercise	No safety concerns reported with about 45 g/day for 6 weeks; safe use of up to 0.42 g/kg body weight (e.g., 30 g/day in a person weighing 154 lb) by many patients with serious conditions (e.g., infections, intestinal diseases, and burns) Reported adverse effects: None known
Iron	Increases oxygen uptake, reduces heart rate, and decreases lactate concentrations during exercise	Numerous clinical trials with conflicting results Research findings: Improved work capacity with correction of iron deficiency anemia; conflicting evidence on whether milder iron deficiency without anemia impairs exercise performance	No safety concerns reported for use at recommended intakes (8 mg/day for healthy men and postmenopausal women and 18 mg/day for healthy premenopausal women) Reported adverse effects: Gastric upset, constipation, nausea, abdominal pain, vomiting, and fainting at intakes above 45 mg/day
Protein	Builds, maintains, and repairs muscle	Numerous clinical trials Research findings: Optimizes muscle training response during exercise and subsequent recovery period	No safety concerns reported at daily recommended intakes for athletes of up to about 2.0 g/kg body weight (e.g., 136 g for a person weighing 150 lb) Reported adverse effects: None known

Table 14.1. Continued

Ingredient	Proposed Mechanism Of Action	Evidence Of Efficacy*	Evidence Of Safety*
Quercetin	Increases mitochondria in muscle, reduces oxidative stress, decreases inflammation, and improves blood flow	Numerous small, short-term clinical trials Research findings: Little to no effect on endurance performance or maximal oxygen consumption	No safety concerns reported for 1,000 mg/day or less for up to 8 weeks Reported adverse effects: None known
Ribose	Involved in production of adenosine triphosphate (ATP)	A few small, short-term, clinical trials Research findings: Little to no effect on exercise capacity in both trained and untrained adults	Safety as a dietary supplement not well studied; no safety concerns reported for up to 10 g/day for 8 weeks Reported adverse effects: None known
Sodium bicarbonate	Enhances disposal of hydrogen ions generated from intense muscle activity, thereby reducing metabolic acidosis and resulting fatigue	Many small, short-term clinical trials Research findings: Might provide minor to moderate performance benefit for short-term and intermittent high-intensity activity, especially in trained athletes	No safety concerns reported for short-term use of up to 300 mg/kg body weight Reported adverse effects: Nausea, stomach pain, diarrhea, and vomiting
Tart or sour cherry	Phytochemicals in tart cherries may facilitate exercise recovery by reducing pain and inflammation	A few clinical trials with conflicting results Research findings: Variable results for aiding muscle strength recovery, reducing soreness, or reducing inflammatory effects on lungs after exercise; insufficient research on ability to improve aerobic performance	No safety concerns reported for about 1/2 quart of juice or 480 mg freeze-dried Montmorency tart-cherry-skin powder per day for up to 2 weeks Reported adverse effects: None known

Table 14.1. Continued

Ingredient	Proposed Mechanism Of Action	Evidence Of Efficacy*	Evidence Of Safety*
Tribulus terrestris	Increases serum testosterone and luteinizing hormone concentrations, thereby promoting skeletal muscle hypertrophy	A few small, short-term clinical trials Research findings: No effect on strength, lean body mass, or sex hormone levels	Safety not well studied; no safety concerns reported at up to 3.21 mg/kg/day for 8 weeks Reported adverse effects: One case report of harm from product labeled but not confirmed to contain *Tribulus terrestris*

The evidence of efficacy and safety is for the individual ingredients. The efficacy and safety of these ingredients might be different when they are combined with other ingredients in a product or training plan.

Part Two
Sports Safety And Injury Prevention

Chapter 15

Healthy Muscles Matter

Basic Facts About Muscles

Did you know you have more than 600 muscles in your body? These muscles help you move, lift things, pump blood through your body, and even help you breathe.

When you think about your muscles, you probably think most about the ones you can control. These are your voluntary muscles, which means you can control their movements. They are also called skeletal muscles, because they attach to your bones and work together with your bones to help you walk, run, pick up things, play an instrument, throw a baseball, kick a soccer ball, push a lawnmower, or ride a bicycle. The muscles of your mouth and throat even help you talk!

Keeping your muscles healthy will help you to be able to walk, run, jump, lift things, play sports, and do all the other things you love to do. Exercising, getting enough rest, and eating a balanced diet will help to keep your muscles healthy for life.

Different Kinds Of Muscles Have Different Jobs

Skeletal muscles are connected to your bones by tough cords of tissue called tendons. As the muscle contracts, it pulls on the tendon, which moves the bone. Bones are connected to other bones by ligaments, which are like tendons and help hold your skeleton together.

Smooth muscles are also called involuntary muscles since you have no control over them. Smooth muscles work in your digestive system to move food along and push waste out of your body. They also help keep your eyes focused without your having to think about it.

About This Chapter: This chapter includes text excerpted from "Healthy Muscles Matter," National Institute of Arthritis and Musculoskeletal and Skin Diseases (NIAMS), October 2015.

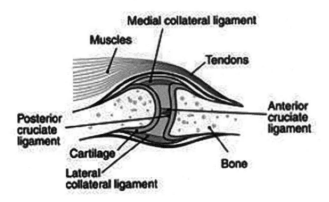

Figure 15.1. A Joint Showing Muscles, Ligaments, And Tendons.

Cardiac muscle. Did you know your heart is also a muscle? It is a specialized type of involuntary muscle. It pumps blood through your body, changing its speed to keep up with the demands you put on it. It pumps more slowly when you're sitting or lying down, and faster when you're running or playing sports and your skeletal muscles need more blood to help them do their work.

Why Healthy Muscles Matter To You

Healthy muscles let you move freely and keep your body strong. They help you to enjoy playing sports, dancing, walking the dog, swimming, and other fun activities. And they help you do those other (not so fun) things that you have to do, like making the bed, vacuuming the carpet, or mowing the lawn.

Strong muscles also help to keep your joints in good shape. If the muscles around your knee, for example, get weak, you may be more likely to injure that knee. Strong muscles also help you keep your balance, so you are less likely to slip or fall.

And remember—the activities that make your skeletal muscles strong will also help to keep your heart muscle strong!

What Can Go Wrong?

Injuries

Almost everyone has had sore muscles after exercising or working too much. Some soreness can be a normal part of healthy exercise. But, in other cases, muscles can become strained.

Muscle strain can be mild (the muscle has just been stretched too much) to severe (the muscle actually tears). Maybe you lifted something that was too heavy and the muscles in your arms were stretched too far. Lifting heavy things in the wrong way can also strain the muscles in your back. This can be very painful and can even cause an injury that will last a long time and make it hard to do everyday things.

The tendons that connect the muscles to the bones can also be strained if they are pulled or stretched too much. If ligaments (remember, they connect bones to bones) are stretched or pulled too much, the injury is called a sprain. Most people are familiar with the pain of a sprained ankle.

Contact sports like soccer, football, hockey, and wrestling can often cause strains. Sports in which you grip something (like gymnastics or tennis) can lead to strains in your hand or forearm.

How Do I Keep My Muscles More Healthy?

Physical Activity

When you make your muscles work by being physically active, they respond by growing stronger. They may even get bigger by adding more muscle tissue. This is how bodybuilders get such big muscles, but your muscles can be healthy without getting that big.

There are lots of activities you can do for your muscles. Walking, jogging, lifting weights, playing tennis, climbing stairs, jumping, and dancing are all good ways to exercise your muscles. Swimming and biking will also give your muscles a good workout. It's important to get different kinds of activities to work all your muscles. And any activity that makes you breathe harder and faster will help exercise that important heart muscle as well!

Get 60 minutes of physical activity every day. It doesn't have to be all at once, but it does need to be in at least 10-minute increments to count toward your 60 minutes of physical activity per day.

Eat A Healthy Diet

You really don't need a special diet to keep your muscles in good health. Eating a balanced diet will help manage your weight and provide a variety of nutrients for your muscles and overall health. A balanced diet:

- Emphasizes fruits, vegetables, whole grains, and fat-free or low-fat dairy products like milk, cheese, and yogurt.

- Includes protein from lean meats, poultry, seafood, beans, eggs, and nuts.

- Is low in solid fats, saturated fats, cholesterol, salt (sodium), added sugars, and refined grains.

- Is as low as possible in *trans* fats.

- Balances calories taken in through food with calories burned in physical activity to help maintain a healthy weight.

As you grow and become an adult, iron is an important nutrient, especially for girls. Not getting enough iron can cause anemia, which can make you feel weak and tired because your muscles don't get enough oxygen. This can also keep you from getting enough activity to keep your muscles healthy. You can get iron from foods like lean beef, chicken and turkey; beans and peas; spinach; and iron-enriched breads and cereals. You can also get iron from dietary supplements, but it's always good to check with a doctor first.

Some people think that supplements will make their muscles bigger and stronger. However, supplements like creatine can cause serious side effects, and protein and amino acid supplements are no better than getting protein from your food. Using steroids to increase your muscles is illegal (unless a doctor has prescribed them for a medical problem), and can have dangerous side effects. No muscle-building supplement can take the place of good nutrition and proper training.

Prevent Injuries

To help prevent sprains, strains, and other muscle injuries:

- Warm up and cool down. Before exercising or playing sports, warm-up exercises, such as stretching and light jogging, may make it less likely that you'll strain a muscle. They are called warm-up exercises because they make the muscles warmer—and more flexible. Cool-down exercises loosen muscles that have tightened during exercise.

- Wear the proper protective gear for your sport, for example pads or helmets. This will help reduce your risk for injuring your muscles or joints.

- Remember to drink lots of water while you're playing or exercising, especially in warm weather. If your body's water level gets too low (dehydration), you could get dizzy or even pass out. Dehydration can cause many medical problems.

- Don't try to "play through the pain." If something starts to hurt, STOP exercising or playing. You might need to see a doctor, or you might just need to rest the injured part for a while.

- If you have been inactive, "start low and go slow" by gradually increasing how often and how long activities are done. Increase physical activity gradually over time.

- Be careful when you lift heavy objects. Keep your back straight and bend your knees to lift the object. This will protect the muscles in your back and put most of the weight on the strong muscles in your legs. Get someone to help you lift something heavy.

Start Now

Keeping your muscles healthy will help you have more fun and enjoy the things you do. Healthy muscles will help you look your best and feel full of energy. Start good habits now, while you are young, and you'll have a better chance of keeping your muscles healthy for the rest of your life.

Chapter 16

The Benefits Of Preseason Conditioning

The number of teens participating in recreational and competitive sports has been steadily on the rise over the past decade. While playing a sport has many physical and mental benefits, teens who lack adequate preparation to handle the demands of the game may not perform to the level they desire and are at greater risk of injury. Poor nutrition, a sedentary lifestyle, and poor physical fitness levels can all stand in the way of being prepared to play.

The gap between deciding to take up a sport and actually competing needs to be bridged by a preparticipation examination and developing a preparatory conditioning program based on the outcome of that exam. This preparatory or preseason conditioning should focus on strength, flexibility, and aerobic training and should be started at least 6 to 8 weeks prior to the competition. For example, if the season starts in June, then the preseason conditioning should start from March or April.

Preparticipation Exam

A preparticipation examination by a physician is needed to identify any risk factors involved in a teen taking up a new sport. Based on their examination, they will be able to identify any underlying conditions or diseases that may need to be addressed, such as asthma or diabetes. The doctor can also assess the physical fitness of the teen and work with them and their parents to create a personalized preseason conditioning program that includes information on the type, intensity, frequency, and duration of the program. The personalized program should also take into account those chronic conditions previously identified, such as anemia, seizures, or asthma.

"The Benefits Of Preseason Conditioning," © 2017 Omnigraphics. Reviewed July 2017.

Preseason Conditioning

The first stage in preseason conditioning is to achieve a high level of overall fitness. Coaches and trainers should not push or engage athletes directly in sport-specific activities at the start of the preseason.

Preseason conditioning should also include exercises to improve the athlete's balance, stabilization, and coordination, which will improve their overall agility. Strengthening exercises for back muscles, especially the core muscles, should be performed to prevent back issues.

As sports-specific skills are introduced into the program, preseason training should also take into account the conditions under which the athlete will be performing. For example, if the sport is played predominately in the summer, the athlete will need to become conditioned to hot temperature, so he or she may be gradually exposed to longer and more strenuous training outdoors.

Any preseason training program should incorporate adequate recovery time so as to avoid injuries and to promote physical development. And the program should be regularly reviewed and modified in order to optimize gains in fitness and prevent overtraining.

Being Safe During Training

Following the below safety measures during preseason training will help make any program a success:

- Know your limits.
- Drink plenty of water.
- Gradual acclimatization to temperature changes (heat and cold), humidity, and altitude.
- Do not overtrain or suddenly increase the load or intensity of training.
- Immediately report any injury or sudden distress (dizziness, shortness of breath, nausea) to a responsible adult.
- Make sure coaches and trainers know of any medications you are currently taking.
- Always warm up and cool down adequately.
- Use protective gear that is properly fitted and of good quality.
- Wear shoes that provide proper stability and support.
- Avoid training on hard surfaces.
- Get to know the rules of the sport and follow them.

Importance Of Preseason Conditioning

Preseason conditioning is an important element of a well-rounded sports program. A well-designed program will make sure a young athlete has overall physical health and strength on and off the field, not just the particular skills they need to play a given sport. Without preseason conditioning, a young adult may quickly become injured or suffer from burnout early in competition. It is the shared responsibility of the athlete, parents, coaches, and trainers to make sure they are prepared for the demands of competition and to perform to the best of their abilities.

References

1. "NCAA Emphasizes Importance Of Preseason Preparation, Conditioning And Acclimatization," National Collegiate Athletic Association (NCAA), August 23, 2013.

2. "Preseason Conditioning For Young Athletes," American College of Sports Medicine (ACSM), n.d.

3. "Pre-Season Training: What Is It And Why Is It Important?" FitnessHealth Ltd., August 24, 2015.

Chapter 17

Warm Up To Work Out

Warming up is an important training component for any sport. A well-designed warm-up routine prepares an athlete physiologically and psychologically. It gradually increases the heart rate and body temperature, loosens joints, and increases the blood flow to the muscles. It stimulates the cardiovascular system, neuromuscular system, respiratory system, and metabolic energy systems.

As you warm up, the body's demand for oxygen increases, the muscles begin to contract and the heart starts to pump out more blood. This increases the blood flow in the blood vessels and delivers it to the working muscle groups. As the blood flow increases, temperature of body and muscle rises. This helps the muscles use glucose and fatty acids to burn calories. As more calories are burned, the muscles produce more energy for more intense activity.

A gradual warm-up increases elasticity of soft tissues like muscles and tendons, and, as the flexibility of these soft tissues increases, the risk of injuries reduces. Joints also loosen, allowing for a fuller range of motion.

As warm-up progresses, the neural system begins to exert better control over the muscles. This improves mental alertness, body awareness, balance, and agility.

Types Of Warm-Ups

Athletes will generally perform two types of warm-ups:

1. General warm-up

2. Specific warm-up

A general warm-up improves the overall functional potential of the young athlete by increasing the core body temperature and blood supply to meet the oxygen demand. The general warm-up also reduces the postexercise muscle soreness and helps the athlete to recover quickly. Aerobic activities like slow jogging or cycling can be included in general warm-up activities.

Stretching exercises are also an important component of a general warm-up routine. Stretching should be done only after the muscles are warmed up. This will ensure a better stretch since the muscles are more flexible and pliable. If stretches are done without warming up, it could result in muscle tears or strains.

A sport-specific warm-up establishes a connection between the general warm-up and the sport being played. After the core body temperature has been elevated and stretches completed, it is time to work on the specific group of muscles that will be used most intensively. More vigorous activity resembling the type of movements and actions involved in the sport should be featured.

Duration And Intensity Of Warm-Ups

The ideal duration and intensity of a warm-up session will depend on nature of the sport, level of competition, and age of the athlete. Generally, athletes are expected to do 15 to 20 minutes of warm-up, with 5 to 10 minutes of general warm-up and another 10 minutes of sports-specific workouts for greater benefits.

Both the duration and intensity can be modified according to the external environmental temperature and what the athlete is wearing. Also, the warm-up should be timed so that it occurs only 15 minutes or less before the start of competition. Otherwise, the heat dissipates and body temperature returns to normal levels.

Become A Better Athlete

Athletes should invest quality time and effort in a warm-up routine. That extra effort will help them perform to their maximum level, become a better athlete, and also avoid injury in the future.

References

1. Cinelli, Mark. "The Importance Of Warming Up Before Activity," Boston Herald, May 8, 2013.

2. "Fit Facts," American Council on Exercise, n.d.

3. Walker, Brad. "Warm Up Exercises And Stretches," The Stretching Institute, May 25, 2017.

Chapter 18

Physical Activities For Strength And Flexibility

Regular physical activity in children and adolescents promotes health and fitness. Compared to those who are inactive, physically active youth have higher levels of cardiorespiratory fitness and stronger muscles. They also typically have lower body fatness. Their bones are stronger, and they may have reduced symptoms of anxiety and depression.

Youth who are regularly active also have a better chance of a healthy adulthood. Children and adolescents don't usually develop chronic diseases, such as heart disease, hypertension, type 2 diabetes, or osteoporosis. However, risk factors for these diseases can begin to develop early in life. Regular physical activity makes it less likely that these risk factors will develop and more likely that children will remain healthy as adults.

Youth can achieve substantial health benefits by doing moderate- and vigorous-intensity physical activity for periods of time that add up to 60 minutes (1 hour) or more each day. This activity should include aerobic activity as well as age-appropriate muscle- and bone-strengthening activities.

Although current science is not complete, it appears that, as with adults, the total amount of physical activity is more important for achieving health benefits than is any one component (frequency, intensity, or duration) or specific mix of activities (aerobic, muscle-strengthening, bone strengthening). Even so, bone-strengthening activities remain especially important for children and young adolescents because the greatest gains in bone mass occur during the years just before and during puberty. In addition, the majority of peak bone mass is obtained by the end of adolescence.

About This Chapter: This chapter includes text excerpted from "Physical Activity Guidelines—Chapter 3: Active Children And Adolescents," Office of Disease Prevention and Health Promotion (ODPHP), U.S. Department of Health and Human Services (HHS), October 7, 2008. Reviewed July 2017.

Here's an example of how to fit 60 minutes of physical activity into your day:

10 minutes—to walk or bike to a friend's house

+

30 minutes—of playing baskaetball

+

10 minutes—of chasing the dog around the yard

+

10 minutes—to walk back home

= 60 minutes of activity!

(Source: "Take Charge Of Your Health: A Guide For Teenagers," National Institute of Diabetes and Digestive and Kidney Diseases (NIDDK).)

This chapter provides physical activity guidance for children and adolescents aged 6 to 17, and focuses on physical activity beyond baseline activity.

Parents and other adults who work with or care for youth should be familiar with the Guidelines. These adults should be aware that, as children become adolescents, they typically reduce their physical activity. Adults play an important role in providing age-appropriate opportunities for physical activity. In doing so, they help lay an important foundation for life-long, health-promoting physical activity. Adults need to encourage active play in children and encourage sustained and structured activity as children grow older.

Key Guidelines For Children And Adolescents

- Children and adolescents should do 60 minutes (1 hour) or more of physical activity daily.

- **Aerobic:** Most of the 60 or more minutes a day should be either moderate- or vigorous-intensity aerobic physical activity, and should include vigorous-intensity physical activity at least 3 days a week.

- **Muscle-strengthening:** As part of their 60 or more minutes of daily physical activity, children and adolescents should include muscle-strengthening physical activity on at least 3 days of the week.

- **Bone-strengthening:** As part of their 60 or more minutes of daily physical activity, children and adolescents should include bone-strengthening physical activity on at least 3 days of the week.

- It is important to encourage young people to participate in physical activities that are appropriate for their age, that are enjoyable, and that offer variety.

Explaining The Guidelines

Types Of Activity

The *Physical Activity Guidelines for Americans* (PAG or the Guidelines) for children and adolescents focus on three types of activity: aerobic, muscle-strengthening, and bone-strengthening. Each type has important health benefits.

- **Aerobic activities** are those in which young people rhythmically move their large muscles. Running, hopping, skipping, jumping rope, swimming, dancing, and bicycling are all examples of aerobic activities. Aerobic activities increase cardiorespiratory fitness. Children often do activities in short bursts, which may not technically be aerobic activities.

- **Muscle-strengthening activities** make muscles do more work than usual during activities of daily life. This is called "overload," and it strengthens the muscles. Muscle-strengthening activities can be unstructured and part of play, such as playing on playground equipment, climbing trees, and playing tug-of-war. Or these activities can be structured, such as lifting weights or working with resistance bands.

- **Bone-strengthening activities** produce a force on the bones that promotes bone growth and strength. This force is commonly produced by impact with the ground. Running, jumping rope, basketball, tennis, and hopscotch are all examples of bone strengthening activities. As these examples illustrate, bone-strengthening activities can also be aerobic and muscle-strengthening.

How Age Influences Physical Activity In Children And Adolescents

Children and adolescents should meet the Guidelines by doing activity that is appropriate for their age. Their natural patterns of movement differ from those of adults. For example, children are naturally active in an intermittent way, particularly when they do unstructured active play. During recess and in their free play and games, children use basic aerobic and bone-strengthening activities, such as running, hopping, skipping, and jumping, to develop movement patterns and skills. They alternate brief periods of moderate- and vigorous-intensity physical activity with brief periods of rest. Any episode of moderate- or vigorous–intensity physical activity, however brief, counts toward the Guidelines.

Children also commonly increase muscle strength through unstructured activities that involve lifting or moving their body weight or working against resistance. Children don't usually do or need formal muscle-strengthening programs, such as lifting weights.

As children grow into adolescents, their patterns of physical activity change. They are able to play organized games and sports and are able to sustain longer periods of activity. But they still commonly do intermittent activity, and no period of moderate- or vigorous-intensity activity is too short to count toward the Guidelines.

Adolescents may meet the Guidelines by doing free play, structured programs, or both. Structured exercise programs can include aerobic activities, such as playing a sport, and muscle-strengthening activities, such as lifting weights, working with resistance bands, or using body weight for resistance (such as push-ups, pull-ups, and sit-ups). Muscle-strengthening activities count if they involve a moderate to high level of effort and work the major muscle groups of the body: legs, hips, back, abdomen, chest, shoulders, and arms.

Levels Of Intensity For Aerobic Activity

Children and adolescents can meet the Guidelines by doing a combination of moderate- and vigorous intensity aerobic physical activities or by doing only vigorous-intensity aerobic physical activities.

Youth should not do only moderate-intensity activity. It's important to include vigorous-intensity activities because they cause more improvement in cardiorespiratory fitness.

The intensity of aerobic physical activity can be defined on either an absolute or a relative scale. Either scale can be used to monitor the intensity of aerobic physical activity:

- **Absolute intensity** is based on the rate of energy expenditure during the activity, without taking into account a person's cardiorespiratory fitness.

- **Relative intensity** uses a person's level of cardiorespiratory fitness to assess level of effort.

Relative intensity describes a person's level of effort relative to his or her fitness. As a rule of thumb, on a scale of 0 to 10, where sitting is 0 and the highest level of effort possible is 10, moderate-intensity activity is a 5 or 6. Young people doing moderate-intensity activity will notice that their hearts are beating faster than normal and they are breathing harder than normal. Vigorous-intensity activity is at a level of 7 or 8. Youth doing vigorous-intensity activity will feel their heart beating much faster than normal and they will breathe much harder than normal.

When adults supervise children, they generally can't ascertain a child's heart or breathing rate. But they can observe whether a child is doing an activity which, based on absolute energy expenditure, is considered to be either moderate or vigorous. For example, a child walking briskly to school is doing moderate-intensity activity. A child running on the playground is doing vigorous-intensity activity. Table 18.1 includes examples of activities classified by absolute intensity. It shows that the same activity can be moderate or vigorous intensity, depending on factors such as speed (for example bicycling slowly or fast).

Table 18.1. Examples Of Moderate- And Vigorous-Intensity Aerobic Physical Activities And Muscle- And Bone-Strengthening Activities For Children And Adolescents

Type Of Physical Activity	Age Group Children	Age Group Adolescents
Moderate– intensity aerobic	• Active recreation, such as hiking, skateboarding, rollerblading • Bicycle riding • Brisk walking	• Active recreation, such as canoeing, hiking, skateboarding, rollerblading • Brisk walking • Bicycle riding (stationary or road bike) • Housework and yard work, such as sweeping or pushing a lawn mower • Games that require catching and throwing, such as baseball and softball
Vigorous– intensity aerobic	• Active games involving running and chasing, such as tag • Bicycle riding • Jumping rope • Martial arts, such as karate • Running • Sports such as soccer, ice or field hockey, basketball, swimming, tennis • Cross-country skiing	• Active games involving running and chasing, such as flag football • Bicycle riding • Jumping rope • Martial arts, such as karate • Running • Sports such as soccer, ice or field hockey, basketball, swimming, tennis • Vigorous dancing • Cross-country skiing

Table 18.1. Continued

Type Of Physical Activity	Age Group Children	Age Group Adolescents
Muscle-strengthening	• Games such as tug-of-war • Modified push-ups (with knees on the floor) • Resistance exercises using body weight or resistance bands • Rope or tree climbing • Sit-ups (curl-ups or crunches) • Swinging on playground equipment/bars	• Games such as tug-of-war • Push-ups and pull-ups • Resistance exercises with exercise bands, weight machines, hand-held weights • Climbing wall • Sit-ups (curl-ups or crunches)
Bone-strengthening	• Games such as hopscotch • Hopping, skipping, jumping • Jumping rope • Running • Sports such as gymnastics, basketball, volleyball, tennis	• Hopping, skipping, jumping • Jumping rope • Running • Sports such as gymnastics, basketball, volleyball, tennis

Note: Some activities, such as bicycling, can be moderate or vigorous intensity, depending upon level of effort

Physical Activity And Healthy Weight

Regular physical activity in children and adolescents promotes a healthy body weight and body composition.

Exercise training in overweight or obese youth can improve body composition by reducing overall levels of fatness as well as abdominal fatness. Research studies report that fatness can be reduced by regular physical activity of moderate to vigorous intensity 3 to 5 times a week, for 30 to 60 minutes.

> About 20 percent of kids between 12 and 19 years old have obesity. But small changes in your eating and physical activity habits may help you reach and stay a healthy weight.
>
> *(Source: "Take Charge Of Your Health: A Guide For Teenagers," National Institute of Diabetes and Digestive and Kidney Diseases (NIDDK).)*

Meeting The Guidelines

American youth vary in their physical activity participation. Some don't participate at all, others participate in enough activity to meet the Guidelines, and some exceed the Guidelines.

One practical strategy to promote activity in youth is to replace inactivity with activity whenever possible. For example, where appropriate and safe, young people should walk or bicycle to school instead of riding in a car. Rather than just watching sporting events on television, young people should participate in age-appropriate sports or games.

- **Children and adolescents who do not meet the Guidelines** should slowly increase their activity in small steps and in ways that they enjoy. A gradual increase in the number of days and the time spent being active will help reduce the risk of injury.

- **Children and adolescents who meet the Guidelines** should continue being active on a daily basis and, if appropriate, become even more active. Evidence suggests that even more than 60 minutes of activity every day may provide additional health benefits.

- **Children and adolescents who exceed the Guidelines** should maintain their activity level and vary the kinds of activities they do to reduce the risk of overtraining or injury.

Children and adolescents with disabilities are more likely to be inactive than those without disabilities. Youth with disabilities should work with their healthcare provider to understand the types and amounts of physical activity appropriate for them. When possible, children and adolescents with disabilities should meet the Guidelines. When young people are not able to participate in appropriate physical activities to meet the Guidelines, they should be as active as possible and avoid being inactive.

Chapter 19

Facts About Protective Equipment

Taking part in sports and recreation activities is an important part of a healthy, physically active lifestyle for kids. But injuries can, and do, occur. More than 2.6 million children 0–19 years old are treated in the emergency department each year for sports and recreation-related injuries.

Thankfully, there are steps that parents can take to help make sure kids stay safe on the field, the court, or wherever they play or participate in sports and recreation activities.

Key Prevention Tips

Gear up. When children are active in sports and recreation, make sure they use the right protective gear for their activity, such as helmets, wrist guards, knee or elbow pads.

Use the right stuff. Be sure that sports protective equipment is in good condition, fits appropriately and is worn correctly all the time—for example, avoid missing or broken buckles or compressed or worn padding. Poorly fitting equipment may be uncomfortable and may not offer the best protection.

Get an action plan in place. Be sure the sports program or school has an action plan that includes information on how to teach athletes ways to lower their chances of getting a concussion and other injuries. Get more concussion safety tips.

About This Chapter: Text in this chapter begins with excerpts from "Sports Safety," Centers for Disease Control and Prevention (CDC), March 14, 2017; Text under the heading "Safety Equipment" is excerpted from "Safety Equipment," girlshealth.gov, Office on Women's Health (OWH), March 27, 2015.

Pay attention to temperature. Allow time for child athletes to gradually adjust to hot or humid environments to prevent heat-related injuries or illness. Parents and coaches should pay close attention to make sure that players are hydrated and appropriately dressed.

Be a good model. Communicate positive safety messages and serve as a model of safe behavior, including wearing a helmet and following the rules.

Safety Equipment

From helmets to shoes, the right equipment can help keep you safe when playing sports or being active. (Don't worry, you don't need to wear all of these things at once—unless you need a cool costume.)

Helmets

Helmets help when there's a risk of falling or getting hit in the head, like in baseball, softball, biking, skiing, horseback riding, skateboarding, and inline skating. Make sure you wear a helmet that is made for the activity you are doing. And make sure you know how it is supposed to fit. In some states, the law says you have to wear a helmet while biking. Bike helmets should come with a special sticker from the U.S. Consumer Product Safety Commission (CPSC).

Special Eye Protection

Special eye protection helps prevent many sports-related eye injuries. Sports that have a high risk of eye injury include basketball, baseball, hockey, and racquet sports. Regular glasses or sunglasses will not keep your eyes safe from injury. If you wear regular glasses, the protective eyewear goes over them. If you wear goggles, they should fit snugly and have cushioning for a comfortable fit. Goggles made from a special material called polycarbonate are extremely strong. Ask your coach or eye doctor what type of eye protection you may need.

Mouth Guards

Mouth guards protect your mouth, teeth, and tongue. They offer protection in soccer, lacrosse, basketball, baseball, cheerleading, and other activities in which you could get hit in the mouth. You can get mouth guards at sport stores or from your dentist.

Pads For Your Wrists, Knees, And Elbows

Pads for your wrists, knees, and elbows can help prevent lots of injuries, including broken bones. They are important for activities such as inline skating, snowboarding, and hockey.

In some sports, like soccer, your coach may require shin guards, which are pads to protect your lower leg.

Shoes

Shoes need to fit well and be right for your sport. Check with your coach or an athletic shoe salesperson about what shoes to wear. Also ask how often they need to be replaced.

Chapter 20

Helmets

Helmets help when there's a risk of falling or getting hit in the head, like in baseball, soft-ball, biking, skiing, horseback riding, skateboarding, and inline skating. Make sure you wear a helmet that is made for the activity you are doing. And make sure you know how it is supposed to fit. In some states, the law says you have to wear a helmet while biking. Bike helmets should come with a special sticker from the U.S. Consumer Product Safety Commission (CPSC).

Why Are Helmets So Important?

For many recreational activities, wearing a helmet can reduce the risk of a severe head injury and even save your life.

How Does A Helmet Protect My Head?

During a typical fall or collision, much of the impact energy is absorbed by the helmet, rather than your head and brain.

Does This Mean That Helmets Prevent Concussions?

No. No helmet design has been proven to prevent concussions. The materials that are used in most of today's helmets are engineered to absorb the high impact energies that can produce

About This Chapter: Text in this chapter begins with excerpts from "Safety Equipment," girlshealth.gov, Office on Women's Health (OWH), July 1, 2015; Text beginning with the heading "Why Are Helmets So Important?" is excerpted from "Which Helmet For Which Activity?" U.S. Consumer Product Safety Commission (CPSC), May 16, 2014; Text beginning with the heading "Child's Or Teen's Helmet Safety" is excerpted from "Heads Up—Helmet Safety," Centers for Disease Control and Prevention (CDC), February 16, 2015.

skull fractures and severe brain injuries. However, these materials have not been proven to counteract the energies believed to cause concussions. Beware of claims that a particular helmet can reduce or prevent concussions.

To protect against concussion injury, play smart. Learn the signs and symptoms of a concussion so that after a fall or collision, you can recognize the symptoms, get proper treatment, and prevent additional injury.

Are All Helmets The Same?

No. There are different helmets for different activities. Each type of helmet is made to protect your head from the kind of impacts that typically are associated with a particular activity or sport. Be sure to wear a helmet that is appropriate for the particular activity you're involved in. Helmets designed for other activities may not protect your head as effectively.

How Can I Tell Which Helmet Is The Right One To Use?

There are safety standards for most types of helmets. Bicycle and motorcycle helmets must comply with mandatory federal safety standards. Helmets for many other recreational activities are subject to voluntary safety standards.

Helmets that meet the requirements of a mandatory or voluntary safety standard are designed and tested to protect the user from receiving a skull fracture or severe brain injury while wearing the helmet. For example, all bicycle helmets manufactured after 1999 must meet the U.S. Consumer Product Safety Commission (CPSC) bicycle helmet standard (16 C.F.R. part 1203); helmets meeting this standard provide protection against skull fractures and severe brain injuries when the helmet is used properly.

The protection that the appropriate helmet can provide is dependent upon achieving a proper fit and wearing it correctly; for many activities, chin straps are specified in the standard, and they are essential for the helmet to function properly. For example, the bicycle standard requires that chin straps be strong enough to keep the helmet on the head and in the proper position during a fall or collision.

Helmets that meet a particular standard will contain a special label or marking that indicates compliance with that standard (usually found on the liner inside of the helmet, on the exterior surface, or attached to the chin strap). Don't rely solely on the helmet's name or appearance, or claims made on the packaging, to determine whether the helmet meets the appropriate requirements for your activity.

Don't choose style over safety. When choosing a helmet, avoid helmets that contain non-essential elements that protrude from the helmet (e.g., horns, Mohawks)—these may look interesting, but they may prevent the helmet's smooth surface from sliding after a fall, which could lead to injury.

Don't add anything to the helmet, such as stickers, coverings, or other attachments that aren't provided with the helmet, as such items can negatively affect the helmet's performance.

Avoid novelty and toy helmets that are made only to look like the real thing; such helmets are not made to comply with any standard and can be expected to offer little or no protection.

Are There Helmets That I Can Wear For More Than One Activity?

Yes, but only a few. For example, you can wear a United States Consumer Product Safety Commission (CPSC)-compliant bicycle helmet while bicycling, recreational in-line skating or roller skating, or riding a kick scooter.

Are There Any Activities For Which One Should Not Wear A Helmet?

Yes. Children should not wear a helmet when playing on playgrounds or climbing trees. If a child wears a helmet during these activities, the helmet's chin strap can get caught on the equipment or tree branches and pose a risk of strangulation. The helmet may also prevent a child's head from moving through an opening that the body can fit through, and entrap the child by his/her head.

How Can I Tell If My Helmet Fits Properly?

A helmet should be both comfortable and snug. Be sure that the helmet is worn so that it is level on your head—not tilted back on the top of your head or pulled too low over your forehead. Once on your head, the helmet should not move in any direction, back-to-front or side-to-side. For helmets with a chin strap, be sure the chin strap is securely fastened so that the helmet doesn't move or fall off during a fall or collision.

If you buy a helmet for a child, bring the child with you so that the helmet can be tested for a good fit. Carefully examine the helmet and the accompanying instructions and safety literature.

What Can I Do If I Have Trouble Fitting The Helmet?

Depending on the type of helmet, you may have to apply the foam padding that comes with the helmet, adjust the straps, adjust the air bladders, or make other adjustments specified by the manufacturer. If these adjustments do not work, consult with the store where you bought the helmet or with the helmet manufacturer. Do not add extra padding or parts, or make any adjustments that are not specifically outlined in the manufacturer's instructions. Do not wear a helmet that does not fit correctly.

Will I Need To Replace A Helmet After An Impact?

That depends on the severity of the impact and whether the helmet was designed to withstand one impact (a single-impact helmet) or more than one impact (a multiple-impact helmet). For example, bicycle helmets are designed to protect against the impact from just a single fall, such as a bicyclist's fall onto the pavement. The foam material in the helmet will crush to absorb the impact energy during a fall or collision. The materials will not protect you again from an additional impact. Even if there are no visible signs of damage to the helmet, you must replace it after such an event.

Other helmets are designed to protect against multiple impacts. Two examples are football and ice hockey helmets. These helmets are designed to withstand multiple impacts of the type associated with the respective activities. However, you may still have to replace the helmet after one severe impact if the helmet has visible signs of damage, such as a cracked shell or permanent dent in the shell or liner. Consult the manufacturer's instructions or certification stickers on the helmet for guidance on when the helmet should be replaced.

How Long Are Helmets Supposed To Last?

Follow the guidance provided by the manufacturer. In the absence of such guidance, it may be prudent to replace your helmet within 5–10 years of purchase, a decision that can be based, at least in part, on how much the helmet was used, how it was cared for, and where it was stored. Cracks in the shell or liner, a loose shell, marks on the liner, fading of the shell, evidence of crushed foam in the liner, worn straps, and missing pads or other parts, are all reasons to replace a helmet. Regular replacement may minimize any reduced effectiveness that could result from degradation of materials over time, and allow you to take advantage of recent advances in helmet protection.

Child's Or Teen's Helmet Safety

A child's helmet should fit properly and be:

- Well maintained

- Age appropriate

- Worn consistently and correctly

- Appropriately certified for use

While there is no concussion-proof helmet, a helmet can help protect the child or teen from a serious brain or head injury. Even with a helmet, it is important for the child or teen to avoid hits to the head.

Batter's Helmet Safety

While there is no concussion-proof helmet, a batter's helmet can help protect your athlete from a serious brain or head injury.

Just For Batters

Check with your athlete's team or league to see if faceguards are required to be worn by athletes when batting. If a faceguard is required, it is important to read the manufacturer's instructions on fit and care. A softball only faceguard should not be used for a baseball player, as the opening on a softball only faceguard is large enough to allow a baseball to come through.

Start With The Right Size—Bring The Athlete

Bring your athlete with you when buying a new helmet to make sure that you can check for a good fit.

Head Size

To find out your athlete's head size, wrap a soft tape measure around the athlete's head, just above their eyebrows and ears. Make sure the tape measure stays level from front to back. (If you don't have a soft tape measure, you can use a string and then measure it against a ruler.)

Sizes Will Vary

Helmet sizes often will vary from brand-to-brand and with different models. Each helmet will fit differently, so it is important to check out the manufacturer's website for the helmet brand's fit instructions and sizing charts, as well as to find out what helmet size fits your athlete's head size.

Get A Good Fit

General Fit

A batter's helmet should fit snugly all around, with no spaces between the pads and the athlete's head. Athletes should NOT wear anything under their batter's helmet, unless recommended by a healthcare professional. This includes a baseball cap. Wearing a baseball cap under the helmet may prevent the helmet from fitting properly.

Ask

Ask your athlete how the helmet feels on their head. While it needs to have a snug fit, a helmet that is too tight can cause headaches.

Hairstyle

An athlete should try on the helmet with the hairstyle he or she will wear for practices and games. Helmet fit can change if the athlete's hairstyle changes considerably. For example, a long-haired player who gets a very short haircut will need to adjust the fit of the helmet.

Coverage

A batter's helmet should not sit too high or low on the athlete's head. To check, make sure the ear holes line up with the athlete's ears. When the athlete is looking straight forward, the bill of the batter's helmet should be parallel to the ground. The bottom of the pad inside the front of the helmet should be one inch above the athlete's eyebrows.

Vision

Make sure you can see the athlete's eyes and that he or she can see straight forward and side-to-side.

Take Care Of The Helmet

Check For Damage

Do not allow your athlete to use a cracked or broken helmet or a helmet that is missing any padding or parts. Check for missing or loose padding before the season and regularly during the season.

Cleaning

Clean the helmet often inside and out with warm water and mild detergent. DO NOT soak any part of the helmet, put it close to high heat, or use strong cleaners.

Protect

Do not let anyone sit or lean on the helmet.

Storage

Do not store a batter's helmet in a car. The helmet should be stored in a room that does not get too hot or too cold and where the helmet is away from direct sunlight.

Decoration

Do not decorate (paint or put stickers on) the helmet without checking with the helmet manufacturer, as this may affect the safety of the helmet. This information may also be found on the instructions label or on the manufacturer's website.

Look For A Batter's Helmet With Labels

- Labels that have the date of manufacture. This information will be helpful in case the helmet is recalled; and

- Labels say National Operating Committee on Standards for Athletic Equipment (NOCSAE®) certified. That label means that the helmet has been tested for safety and meets the federal safety standards.

If the helmet is not new, you should also look for a label that includes the date the helmet was expertly repaired and approved for use (reconditioned/recertified). Helmets that have been properly reconditioned and recertified will have a label with the date of recertification and the name of the reconditioning company.

Know When To Replace A Batter's Helmet

Check The Label

Be sure to follow safety labels on the helmet on when to replace the helmet. Some batter's helmets have a label that says that it should not be reconditioned. Helmets with this label will also include how long the helmet can be used. However, some of these helmets may need to be replaced sooner, depending upon wear and tear.

Reconditioning

Reconditioning involves having an expert inspect and repair a used helmet by: fixing cracks or damage, replacing missing parts, testing it for safety, and recertifying it for use. Helmets should be reconditioned regularly by a licensed National Athletic Equipment Reconditioner Association (NAERA)-member. DO NOT allow your athlete to use a used helmet that is not approved/recertified for use by a NAERA reconditioner.

Catcher's Helmet Safety

Start With The Right Size

Bring The Athlete

Bring your athlete with you when buying a new helmet to make sure that you can check for a good fit.

Head Size

To find out the size of your athlete's head, wrap a soft tape measure around the athlete's head, just above their eyebrows and ears. Make sure the tape measure stays level from front to back. (If you don't have a soft tape measure, you can use a string and then measure it against a ruler.)

Sizes Will Vary

Helmet sizes often will vary from brand-to-brand and with different models. Each helmet will fit differently, so it is important to check out the manufacturer's website for the helmet brand's fit instructions and sizing charts, as well as to find out what helmet size fits your athlete's head size.

Get A Good Fit

General Fit

No matter which style of catcher's helmet is used, the helmet should fit snugly all around, with no spaces between the pads and the athlete's head. Athletes should NOT wear anything under their catcher's helmet, unless recommended by a healthcare professional. This includes a baseball cap. Wearing a baseball cap under the helmet may prevent the helmet from fitting properly.

110

Ask

Ask your athlete how the helmet feels on their head. While it needs to have a snug fit, a helmet that is too tight can cause headaches.

Hairstyle

An athlete should try on the helmet with the hairstyle he or she will wear for practices and games. Helmet fit can change if the athlete's hairstyle changes. For example, a long-haired player who gets a very short haircut will need to adjust the fit of the helmet.

Coverage

A catcher's helmet should not sit too high or low on their head. To check, make sure the catcher's mask rests flat on the front of the catcher's helmet. For the two-piece style catcher's helmet, you can tighten or loosen the straps on the sides and top of the face mask to adjust how tightly they grip the helmet.

Vision

Make sure you can see the athlete's eyes and that he or she can see straight forward and side-to-side.

Take Care Of The Helmet

Check For Damage

DO NOT allow your athlete to use a cracked or broken helmet or a helmet that is missing any padding or parts. Check for missing or loose parts or padding before the

season and regularly during the season. Be sure to replace face masks if they are bent.

Cleaning

Clean the helmet often inside and out with warm water and mild detergent. DO NOT soak any part of the helmet, put it close to high heat, or use strong cleaners.

Protect

DO NOT let anyone sit or lean on the helmet.

Storage

Do not store a catcher's helmet in a car. The helmet should be stored in a room that does not get too hot or too cold and where the helmet is away from direct sunlight.

Decoration

DO NOT decorate (paint or put stickers on) the helmet without checking with the helmet manufacturer, as this may affect the safety of the helmet. This information may also be found on the instructions label or on the manufacturer's website.

Look For The Labels

Look For A Catcher's Helmet With Labels That

- Have the date of manufacture. This information will be helpful in case the helmet is recalled.
- Say NOCSAE® certified. That label means that the helmet has been tested for safety and meets safety standards.

If the helmet is not new, you should also look for a label that includes the date the helmet was expertly repaired and approved for use (reconditioned/recertified). Helmets that have been properly reconditioned and recertified will have a label with the date of recertification and the name of the reconditioning company.

When To Replace A Catcher's Helmet

Check The Label

Be sure to follow safety labels on the helmet on when to replace the helmet. Some catcher's helmets have a label that says that it should not be reconditioned. Helmets with this label will also include how long the helmet can be used. However, some of these helmets may need to be replaced sooner, depending upon wear and tear.

Reconditioning

Reconditioning involves having an expert inspect and repair a used helmet by: fixing cracks or damage, replacing missing parts, testing it for safety, and recertifying it for use. Helmets should be reconditioned regularly by a licensed NAERA-member. DO NOT allow your athlete to use a used helmet that is not approved/recertified for use by a NAERA reconditioner.

Football Helmet Safety: Start With The Right Size

Bring The Athlete

Bring your athlete with you when buying a new helmet to make sure that you can check for a good fit.

Head Size

To find out the size of your athlete's head, wrap a soft tape measure around the athlete's head, just above their eyebrows and ears. Make sure the tape measure stays level from front to back. (If you don't have a soft tape measure, you can use a string and then measure it against a ruler.)

Sizes Will Vary

Helmet sizes often will vary from brand-to-brand and with different models. Each helmet will fit differently, so it is important to check out the manufacturer's website for the helmet brand's fit instructions and sizing charts, as well as to find out what helmet size fits your athlete's head size.

Get A Good Fit

General Fit

A football helmet should feel snug with no spaces between the pads and the athlete's head. The helmet should not slide on the head with the chin strap in place. If the helmet can be removed while the chin strap is in place, then the fit is too loose. Some helmets have a unique fitting system or use an air bladder system that requires inflation with a special needle to avoid puncturing the air bladders.

Ask

Ask your athlete how the helmet feels on their head. While it needs to have a snug fit, a helmet that is too tight can cause headaches.

Hairstyle

Your athlete should try on the helmet with the hairstyle he will wear while at practices and games. Helmet fit can change if your athlete's hairstyle changes. For example, a long-haired athlete who gets a very short haircut may need to adjust the fit of the helmet.

Coverage

A football helmet should not sit too high or low on their head. To check, make sure ear holes line up with athlete's ears, and helmet pad covers athlete's head from middle of his forehead to back of his head.

Vision

Make sure you can see your athlete's eyes and that he can see straight forward and side-to-side.

Chin Straps

The chin strap should be centered under the athlete's chin and fit snugly. Tell your athlete to open their mouth wide...big yawn! The helmet should pull down on their head. If not, the chin strap needs to be tighter. Once the chin strap is fastened, the helmet should not move in any direction, back-to-front or side-to-side.

Take Care Of The Helmet

Check For Damage

DO NOT allow your athlete to use a cracked or broken helmet or a helmet that is missing any padding or parts. For air bladder-equipped helmets, make sure to check for proper inflation. DO NOT alter, remove or replace padding or internal parts unless supervised by a trained equipment manager. Check for missing or loose parts and padding before the season and regularly during the season.

Cleaning

Clean the helmet often inside and out with warm water and mild detergent. DO NOT soak any part of the helmet, put it close to high heat, or use strong cleaners.

Protect

DO NOT let anyone sit or lean on the helmet.

Storage

Do not store a football helmet in a car. The helmet should be stored in a room that does not get too hot or too cold and where the helmet is away from direct sunlight.

Decoration

DO NOT decorate (paint or put stickers on) the helmet without checking with the helmet manufacturer, as this may affect the safety of the helmet. This information may also be found on the instructions label or on the manufacturer's website.

Look For A Football Helmet With Labels That

- Have the date of manufacture. This information will be helpful in case the helmet is recalled; and

- Say NOCSAE® certified. That label means that the helmet has been tested for safety and meets safety standards.

If the helmet is not new, you should also look for a label that includes the date the helmet was expertly repaired and approved for use (reconditioned/recertified). Helmets that have been properly reconditioned and recertified will have a label with the date of recertification and the name of the reconditioning company.

Know When To Replace A Football Helmet

Reconditioning

Reconditioning involves having an expert inspect and repair a used helmet by: fixing cracks or damage, replacing missing parts, testing it for safety, and recertifying it for use. Helmets should be reconditioned regularly by a licensed NAERA-member. DO NOT allow your athlete to use a used helmet that is not approved/recertified for use by a NAERA reconditioner.

10 And Out

Football helmets should be replaced no later than 10 years from the date of manufacture. Many helmets will need to be replaced sooner, depending upon wear and tear.

Bike Helmets Safety

Start With The Right Size

Bring The Bike Rider

Children or teens can accompany when elders buy a new helmet for you to make sure that you can check for a good fit.

Head Size

Children or teens can find out the size of their head by wrapping a soft tape measure around his or her head, just above their eyebrows and ears. Make sure the tape measure stays level from front to back. (If you don't have a soft tape measure, you can use a string and then measure it against a ruler.)

Sizes Will Vary

Helmet sizes often will vary from brand-to-brand and with different models. Each helmet will fit differently, so it is important to check out the manufacturer's website for the helmet brand's fit instructions and sizing charts, as well as to find out what helmet size fits the child's or teen's head size.

Get A Good Fit

General Fit

The helmet should fit snugly all around, with no spaces between the foam and bike rider's head.

Ask

Children or teens must be asked on how the helmet feels on their head. While it needs to have a snug fit, a helmet that is too tight can cause headaches.

Hairstyle

Bike helmets are available for riders with long hair. The child or teen should try on the helmet with the hairstyle he or she will wear while bike riding. Helmet fit can change if the child's or teen's hairstyle changes. For example, a long-haired bike rider who gets a very short haircut may need to adjust the fit of the helmet.

Adjustments

Some bike helmets have removable padding or a universal fit ring that can be adjusted to get a good fit.

Coverage

A bike helmet should not sit too high or low on the rider's head. To check, make sure the bottom of the pad inside the front of the helmet is one or two finger widths above the bike rider's eyebrows. The back of the helmet should not touch the top of the bike rider's neck.

Vision

Children and teens must make sure they can see their guardian's eyes that they can see straight forward and side-to-side

Side Straps

The side straps should make a "V" shape under, and slightly in front of, the bike rider's ears.

Chin Straps

The chin strap should be centered under the bike rider's chin and fit snugly, so that no more than one or two fingers fit between the chin and the strap. Children or teens should open their mouth wide…big yawn! The helmet should pull down on their head. If not, the chin strap needs to be tighter. If needed, you can pull the straps from the back of the helmet to adjust the chin straps. Once the chin strap is fastened, the helmet should not move in any direction, back-to-front or side-to-side.

Take Care Of The Helmet

Check For Damage

DO NOT allow your bike rider to use a cracked or broken helmet or a helmet that is missing any padding or parts.

Cleaning

Clean the helmet often inside and out with warm water and mild detergent. DO NOT soak any part of the helmet, put it close to high heat, or use strong cleaners.

Protect

DO NOT let anyone sit or lean on the helmet.

Storage

Do not store a bike helmet in a car. The helmet should be stored in a room that does not get too hot or too cold and where the helmet is away from direct sunlight.

Decoration

DO NOT decorate (paint or put stickers on) the helmet without checking with the helmet manufacturer, as this may affect the safety of the helmet. This information may also be found on the instructions label or on the manufacturer's website.

Look For A Bike Helmet With Labels That

- Have the date of manufacture. This information will be helpful in case the helmet is recalled; and

- Say U.S. Consumer Product Safety Commission (CPSC) certified. That label means that the helmet has been tested for safety and meets the federal safety standard.

Some bike helmets may also have a label stating that they are ASTM, Snell, or ANSI certified. These labels let you know that the helmet has also passed the safety tests of these organizations.

When To Replace A Bike Helmet

One Impact

Replace any bicycle helmet that is damaged or has been involved in a crash. Bicycle helmets are designed to help protect the rider's brain and head from one serious impact, such as a fall onto the pavement. You may not be able to see the damage to the foam, but the foam materials in the helmet will crush after an impact. That means that the foam in the helmet won't be able to help protect the rider's brain and head from another impact.

Multi-Use Helmets

Some helmet companies have created multi-use helmets for biking, skateboarding, and other activities. Multi-use helmets are designed to withstand multiple very minor hits; however, a multi-use helmet MUST be replaced if it has been involved in a serious crash or is damaged. Before the child or teen uses a multi-use helmet for biking, make sure the helmet has a CPSC label certifying it for biking.

Chapter 21

Eye Protection

Eye injuries are the leading cause of blindness in children in the United States and most injuries occurring in school-aged children are sports-related. These injuries account for an estimated 100,000 physician visits per year at a cost of more than $175 million.

Ninety percent of sports-related eye injuries can be avoided with the use of protective eyewear. Protective eyewear includes safety glasses and goggles, safety shields, and eye guards designed for a particular sport. Ordinary prescription glasses, contact lenses, and sunglasses do not protect against eye injuries. Safety goggles should be worn over them.

Currently, most youth sports leagues do not require the use of eye protection. Parents and coaches must insist that children wear safety glasses or goggles whenever they play.

Protective eyewear, which is made of ultra-strong polycarbonate, is 10 times more impact resistant than other plastics, and does not reduce vision. All children who play sports should use protective eyewear-not just those who wear eyeglasses or contact lenses. For children who do wear glasses or contact lenses, most protective eyewear can be made to match their pre-scriptions. It is especially important for student athletes who have vision in only one eye or a history of eye injury or eye surgery to use protective eyewear.

Whether you are a parent, teacher, or coach, you can encourage schools to adopt a policy on protective eyewear. Meanwhile, parents and coaches should insist that children wear protective eyewear whenever they play sports and be good role models and wear it themselves.

About This Chapter: This chapter includes text excerpted from "About Sports Eye Injury And Protective Eyewear," National Eye Institute (NEI), April 5, 2017.

Protective Eyewear Fast Facts

- Everyone should wear protective eyewear.
- Ordinary prescription glasses, contact lenses, and sunglasses won't protect you from injuries. Most protective eyewear can be made to match your prescription.
- For the best protection, use eyewear made of ultra-strong polycarbonate.
- Choose eyewear specifically made for your sport and make sure it fits comfortably on your face.

(Source: "Sports And Your Eyes," National Eye Institute (NEI).)

Sport-Specific Risk

Some sports carry a greater risk than others. For example, baseball is the leading cause of sports-related eye injury in children 14 and under and is considered high risk. Football carries a moderate risk.

Finding The Appropriate Eye Protection

The following table summarizes recommended eye protection for a variety of sports. Visit your eye care professional or local sporting goods store to learn more about the most appropriate type of protective eyewear for the child and to ensure proper fit.

Table 21.1. Sport And Its Appropriate Eye Protection

Sport	Eye Protection
Badminton	Sports goggles with polycarbonate lenses
Baseball	Polycarbonate face guard or other certified safe protection attached to the helmet for batting and base running; sports goggles with polycarbonate lenses for fielding
Basketball	Sports goggles with polycarbonate lenses
Bicycling (LER)	Sturdy street-wear frames with polycarbonate or CR-39 lenses
Boxing	None is available
Fencing	Full-face cage
Field Hockey (both sexes)	Goalie: full-face mask; all others: sports goggles with polycarbonate lenses
Football	Polycarbonate shield on helmet

Table 21.1. Continued

Sport	Eye Protection
Full-contact martial arts	Not allowed
Handball	Sports goggles with polycarbonate lenses
Ice Hockey	Helmet and full-face protection
Lacrosse (male)	Helmet and full-face protection required
Lacrosse (female)	Should at least wear sports goggles with polycarbonate lenses and have option to wear helmet and full-face protection
Racquetball	Sports goggles with polycarbonate lenses
Soccer	Sports goggles with polycarbonate lenses
Softball	Polycarbonate face guard on a helmet for batting and base running; sports goggles with polycarbonate lenses for fielding
Squash	Sports goggles with polycarbonate lenses
Street hockey	Sports goggles with polycarbonate lenses; goalie: full face cage
Swimming and pool sports	Swim goggles recommended
Tennis: doubles	Sports goggles with polycarbonate lenses
Tennis: singles	Sturdy street-wear frames with polycarbonate lenses
Track and field (LER)	Sturdy street-wear frames with polycarbonate or CR-39 lenses
Water polo	Swim goggles with polycarbonate lenses
Wrestling	None is available

First Aid Tips

If particles, like sand or dust, get into your eyes, don't rub! Wash your eyes out with water.

If you get hit in the eye with a ball, rock, or elbow, gently put a cold compress on your eye for 15 minutes. This should make the swelling go down and relieve the pain. Have an adult take you to the doctor.

If a chemical from a class experiment, cleaning fluid, or battery acid splashes in your eye, wash your eye out with water for at least 10 minutes. Have an adult take you to the doctor immediately.

If an object like a stick or pencil gets stuck in your eye, don't pull it out. This is very serious. Have an adult put a loose bandage on your eye. Don't put any pressure on the object. Have an adult take you to the doctor immediately.

(Source: "First Aid Tips," National Eye Institute (NEI).)

Chapter 22

Bracing And Taping

Bracing and taping are methods of wrapping that provide support to muscles, tendons, and ligaments and prevent injuries such as sprains, strains, and fractures. Bracing and taping also helps reduce the risk of re-injury when a player goes back out on the field. Ankle sprains account for 2 million sports injuries annually. Most athletes and coaches are familiar with ankle bracing and taping and routinely apply it before every game.

What Is Bracing?

Braces are suitable for athletes who require additional support following an injury. They have solid pieces of polymer or metal and can be adjusted during practice and competition. Braces are designed to enhance mobility rather than immobilize the affected area. A safe degree of movement allows bones and ligaments to heal better. Braces can also help athletes extend physical therapy by allowing them to perform strengthening exercises on their own.

What Is Taping?

Athletic tape is self-adhesive and is used to maintain muscle and bone alignment by limiting excessive movement of the ligaments and joints. Tapes are available in various strengths and colors, with different properties including levels of flexibility and moisture-wicking ability. For optimum effect, taping should be done by a professional doctor, trainer, or physical therapist since incorrectly taping will only worsen the injury. The most significant issue with taping is that it is a temporary fix. The binding power of tape lessens due to sweat and movement. The endurance of tape will last for not more than 30 minutes with continuous sports activity.

"Bracing And Taping," © 2017 Omnigraphics. Reviewed July 2017.

What Are The Differences Between Bracing And Taping?

Braces have a significant advantage over tape because they can be applied, used, and adjusted by athletes without the need for professional help.

Many studies have been conducted on the effectiveness of taping and bracing. Among the findings:

- It has been definitively established that bracing and taping offers significant benefits as compared to not using either.

- Tapes last only for 3 to 4 days before becoming ineffective while braces can help keep your active lifestyle.

- While compression can help with injury management, excessive compression can cause problems.

- Braces are more cost effective than tapes in the long run. In a competitive season, taping is three times more expensive than bracing.

- Athletes feel less comfortable and stable wearing braces than tapes.

- Sweating when exercising and playing sports affects the position of tapes and causes tapes to slip. Braces, on the other hand, cover a larger area and can be adjusted manually. Braces are made of breathable material and allow perspiration without affecting its position.

- Applying taping incorrectly can render it ineffective or may even lead to blistering. Braces can be applied easily and effectively without much reason for concern.

- The choice of tapes or braces depends on preference and experience.

How Does Bracing And Taping Decrease The Severity Of Injuries In Athletes?

Various studies have been conducted on how bracing and taping helps prevent injury and the incidence of reinjury. One theory suggests that bracing and taping increases proprioception, which is the body's unconscious ability to sense affected body part, in athletes. The traction or pressure on skin due to bracing and taping improves sensory input and proprioception where it is in space and in what direction and how fast it is moving. However, recent research also seems to indicate that wrapping actually reduces proprioceptive feedback.

Another study indicated that wearing high top shoes with taping resulted in 50 percent less injuries as compared to wearing low top shoes along with taping.

References

1. Reeves, Douglas A. "Ankle Taping and Bracing," WebMD LLC., June 12, 2017.

2. Hamel, Andrea. "Sports Taping Vs. Bracing – Which Is Right for Your Injury?" Mueller Sports Medicine, Inc., June 2, 2016.

3. "To Tape or To Brace... Is That the question?" Nationwide Children's Hospital, n.d.

4. "Ankle Injuries: To Tape or Not to Tape?" Minnesota Sports Medicine (MSM), n.d.

Chapter 23

How To Select The Right Clothes And Shoes

What To Wear To Work Out

Wondering what to wear when you work out? Well, lots of activities don't require any special clothes. Sometimes, your clothes do matter.

Choosing Workout Clothes

When picking a workout outfit, remember:

- **Don't wear clothes that are very tight.** You need to be able to move freely. And if you want to stay cool, air needs to reach your skin so it can dry your sweat.

- **Color matters (really).** In the summer, lighter colors will help you keep cooler. In the winter, dark clothes trap light and help you stay warm.

- **Wear layers when it is cold out.** You can take some off as you warm up.

- **Think about your head.** Wear a hat or cap for sun protection. In cold weather, wear wool or ski caps to stay warm.

- **Find the right fabric.** If you are going to sweat, you may be more comfortable in material that soaks up wetness. Try a synthetic, like polypropylene. Cotton may be less comfortable because it stays wet longer.

- **Consider wearing a comfortable sports bra.** Wearing a supportive sports bra can help protect your breasts and keep them from bouncing painfully while exercising. Try on a

About This Chapter: This chapter includes text excerpted from "What To Wear To Work Out," girlshealth.gov, Office on Women's Health (OWH), March 27, 2015.

few to see which style you prefer. If you need help finding the right fit, ask for help in a department store or bra store.

How To Pick The Right Workout Shoes

Wearing the right shoes when you work out is very important. To find the right pair, follow these tips:

- **Make sure your shoes protect your feet.** They should be sturdy and have cushioned soles. They should also have arch supports (the raised part inside that curves under the bottom of your foot).

- **Make sure the shoe is right for what you do.** If you plan to run or play a certain sport a lot, consider shoes made for that activity. Tennis players should wear tennis shoes and runners should wear running shoes, for example. Ask a sports shoe salesperson for help.

- **Get the right fit.** Ask a salesperson to measure your foot and then to check the fit. The wrong fit can hurt or even cause foot problems. Try to shop at the end of the day when your feet are a little larger (just like they are when you exercise). Also, when trying on shoes, wear the kind of socks you wear to work out.

Check your shoes regularly and replace them when they're worn out. You need new shoes when:

- The tread is worn out
- Your feet feel tired after activity
- Your shins, knees, or hips hurt after activity

(Source: "Fitness Shoes And Clothes," Go4Life, National Institutes of Health (NIH).)

Don't use any type running shoes for other sports, as they are not made for lateral movements, making ankle sprains more likely. They also last longer and maintain cushioning better if only used for running. Use only good quality court shoes or cross-trainers for other conditioning activities. Wrestling shoes are recommended for defensive tactics training on matted floors.

(Source: "Starting A Running Program," U.S. Customs and Border Protection (CBP).)

Chapter 24

Safety Tips For Popular Sports

Sports offer immense physical, social, and emotional benefits. However, such benefits can be enjoyed only if teens are healthy enough to play and are not relegated to the sidelines after sustaining an injury. By following safety precautions and being aware of what is happening around them on the field, teens will be able to compete and have fun playing any sport they choose.

General Sports Safety Tips

The guidelines outlined below are applicable to any sports teens play.

Preparation Prior To Playing A Sport

- Before playing any organized sport, you should undergo a preparticipation physical exam (PPE) conducted by a medical practitioner and have your medical history reviewed.

- Fitness level is an important part of the preparation. A healthy diet and proper exercise give you stamina to play harder and longer on the field, and reduce the risk of injury.

- Be sure to warm up before actual play. Jumping jacks, jogging in place, and muscle stretches will help prepare your body for competition.

- Keep yourself hydrated with fluids before, after, and at proper intervals during the game. This is all the more crucial during hot weather.

- Understand the game inside and out. Be aware of:

  - rules you need to follow;

"Safety Tips For Popular Sports," © 2017 Omnigraphics. Reviewed July 2017.

- the use of proper technique; and

- illegal maneuvers that will increase the risk of injury.

- Learn what is happening around you during competition and keep your head up. In certain games, this could be crucial to avoid colliding with another player, which can result in injury, especially in sports where players wear protective head gear. If injured, do not continue to play with pain. It is better to continue playing long term after proper medical intervention than risk it all for the sake of one game. If you continue to play, you risk making the injury worse and being sidelined for a longer period of time.

- Play fair and do not become angry on the field. Allow referees or coaches to handle disputes.

- Make sure one or more responsible adults and first aid are on hand to deal with injuries sustained on the field.

- Make sure your coach has your emergency contact information.

Use Of Protective Gear

The use of appropriate and well-fitting safety equipment and protective gear cannot be emphasized enough in the prevention of sports injuries. Helmets are an essential piece of safety gear in quite a number of sports. They should fit snugly and allow unhindered view on all sides.

Ask your coach about the best equipment available for the sport you are playing. Choose from the best available options for support, padding, helmets, mouth guards, protective eye-wear, and athletic cups. Choose protective equipment that is certified and approved by organizations that govern the sport you play. For instance, the National Operating Committee on Standards for Athletic Equipment (NOCSAE) sets the standards for helmets, facemasks, and shinguards. It is also important to take care of your equipment on an ongoing basis to keep yourself safe. If your helmet is dented or cracked, purchase a new one for adequate safety.

Inspecting Playing Fields And Surfaces

Before a game or practice session begins, inspect the playing surface or field for objects that are likely to cause injury, like shards of glass or other debris. Make note of uneven surfaces, irregularities, and holes or ruts in the ground that could cause ankle sprains or other injuries. If you are playing at night, play in areas that are well lit and safe.

Commitment To Safety

When teens play sports, they should do so under the supervision of qualified adults. Teens should choose to join leagues and teams that are committed to the safety of its players. Play under coaches who foster a spirit of sportsmanship and who think winning and losing are part of the game. A coach who is obsessed with winning might encourage teens to play with an injury, which is not recommended. Also, coaches should have first-hand knowledge of how to administer first aid and cardiopulmonary resuscitation (CPR) techniques. Finally, teens should choose to play sports that match their physique, skill level, and emotional maturity.

Popular Sports Safety Tips

Football

One of the most popular sports in high schools, football is also the leading cause of injury in school sports. Common injuries sustained include ankle sprains, concussions, and injuries to knees and shoulders.

Safety Precautions To Follow

- Football requires a lot of protective gear. Make sure you are geared up sufficiently. At minimum, you should be wearing a helmet, leg and shoulder pads, shoes, mouthguard, and athletic supporter with cup. Consider additional protective gear such as padded neck rolls, forearm pads, gloves, and a flak jacket. If you are wearing glasses, make sure they are made of plastic or shatterproof glass.

- Warm up before the game with jumping jacks, jogging in place, and dynamic stretching.

- Obey the rules of the game and do not try illegal maneuvers. They are risky for you and your opponent.

- Football is a chaotic sport so it is essential to stay aware of where you are and what is happening around you in the field. Paying attention helps you avoid accidental collisions.

- If someone is trying to injure you deliberately, do not confront them. Inform the referee instead.

- Stop playing at the sound of the whistle. It is common for players to get hurt when they become aggressive after the play is called.

Track And Field

Track and field events are great sports for teens and cover a wide range of competition, including sprinting, throwing, and jumping.

Safety Precautions To Follow

- Wear appropriate clothing and shoes when running and remove any jewelry.

- Do not crowd the running track.

- Be considerate of other runners using the track.

- Be conscious that synthetic tracks can become slippery when wet.

- Move away from the inside lanes when you are finished.

- The infield is used for throwing events. Do not cross the infield even when there isn't any event taking place.

- When training or competing off the track, keep the following safety tips in mind. Avoid roads and use footpaths when possible. Use light, bright, and reflective clothing when running in the night. Face oncoming traffic even if you are running on pavement.

- Do not cross hurdles from the landing side.

- Ensure throwing areas for discus, shot put, and hammer throws are dry and clear of foreign objects.

Baseball

Baseball is a relatively safe sport, but the risk of injury exists nevertheless from wild pitching, balls that come off the bat, and on-the-field collisions.

Safety Precautions To Follow

- Wear protective equipment on the field.

  - A helmet should be worn when batting, waiting for a turn to bat, and when running the bases. Helmets should fit snugly and the chin strap must be fastened.

  - A catcher should always wear all recommended safety gear in the game, bullpen or during warm-ups.

  - Baseball spikes should have molded plastic cleats and not metal ones.

  - All players should wear athletic supporters.

- Avoid collisions on the field when focusing on fielding the ball by calling out to other players to back away.

- Follow best practices in the game to avoid injury.

- When batting, learn how to avoid the ball if it is about to hit you. The best way is to turn away from the pitcher, exposing your back and rear instead of your face and midsection.

- Learn how to slide correctly. It is illegal in some leagues to slide head first because of the risk of head injuries and facial cuts.

- Pitching stresses joints and tendons and excessive pitching can result in injuries to wrists, elbows, rotator cuffs, tendons, and ligaments. Adhere to league guidelines that allow you to pitch only for a limited number of innings. This keeps the arms of pitchers in good condition.

Basketball

Basketball is a way of life for millions of American kids. Even though it's a fun sport and a great way to exercise, basketball is nevertheless a contact sport and injuries are common. Basketball injuries are rarely life threatening but injuries such as sprains, bruises, broken fingers and bones, bloody noses, poked eyes, concussions, and ligament tears commonly occur.

Safety Precautions To Follow

- Pay attention to what you wear. A good pair of athletic sneakers with high-top, low-rise, and non-skid sole are the best. Gear up with an athletic supporter, mouthguard, and ankle and wrist braces. If you wear glasses, make sure it is made of plastic or shatterproof glass.

- Clear obstacles from the boundaries of the court, including balls, gym bags, and other gear.

- Avoid collisions by being aware of where your teammates and opponents are at all times.

- Obey the rules of the game and avoid shoving, tripping, or holding. Most injuries can be avoided if you do not commit fouls and obey the referee.

- Know where the ball is. Getting hit with the ball when you are not looking is a common cause of injury. Basketballs are hard enough to break a nose or finger.

Boxing

Boxing is a sport that by its nature can be very dangerous. A punch to the head can cause brain trauma and tissue damage. A majority of injures in boxing stem from a punch to the head.

Safety Precautions To Follow

- Keep your hands wrapped up and wear protective gloves that fit properly and firmly.

- Wear head gear to protect from hard hits that could cause concussions.

- Wear a mouthguard to protect your mouth and teeth.

- Use an abdomen guard to protect the genital area.

- Girls should wear chest protection during training and matches.

- Use shoes that have advanced gripping soles.

Soccer

Soccer is the world's most popular sport. It is easy for kids to learn and a great way to exercise. Soccer is a fast-paced sport that is exciting and fun to play. Soccer is a contact sport and injuries due to on-field collisions are very likely. Minor bruises, ankle sprains, hamstring or calf strains, groin injuries, and concussions are the common sports injuries.

Safety Precautions To Follow

- Protective gear is minimal in soccer. Make sure you are using shoes with molded cleats or ribbed soles. Extra traction is critical when playing in wet or grassy fields. Cleats should fit properly and you should be tightly laced up. Use shin guards fitting snugly around the ankle bone. When buying shinguards, bring your socks and cleats along to check if they fit correctly. Use a mouthguard. The goalies must wear adequate padding and special gloves for stopping shots.

- Before you play, take care of the following:

  - Inspect the field for holes, obstacles, debris, or broken glass.

  - Warm up with jumping jacks, running in place, and dynamic stretching.

  - Inspect the goal post. Make sure they're anchored properly to the ground and the poles are padded to prevent injury in case of collisions.

  - Use nonabsorbent synthetic balls when playing in wet conditions. Leather balls become waterlogged and heavy that could lead to injury.

- While you are playing, take care of the following.

  - Obey the rules of the game.

- Be aware of where your teammates and opponents are during play and keep your head up. Collisions are more likely if you go charging down the field without knowing where the other players are.

- Learn to play with proper technique when heading the ball. Otherwise, you could injure your neck and head.

- Keep your mouth closed and tongue inside your teeth to avoid biting your tongue.

Volleyball

Even though volleyball is considered a relatively safe sport, injuries do happen in this sport as well. Sprains and strains to the ankle, repetitive stress injuries of the knee and shoulder, jammed fingers, bone dislocations, and torn tendons are common injures in volleyball.

Safety Precautions To Follow

- Gear up with knee pads, padded shorts, braces, shoes, mouthguards, athletic cups, and sunglasses or goggles.

- Before you play, take care of the following:

  - Inspect the sand, and confirm that it is not too hot.

  - Clear the playing field of debris and other obstacles so that you do not end up tripping.

  - Warm up with not just a few rounds of serve and volley but with jumping jacks, jogging and dynamic stretching.

- While you are playing, take care of the following:

  - When playing close to the net, do not step over the line on to the opponent's side of the court. Most ankle sprains happen when a player lands on an opponent's foot.

  - Do not hang on to the net post or tug at it. It could fall on the players.

  - Call out to your teammates aloud when you're going to field the ball to avoid colliding with them.

  - Use proper technique when spiking or blocking. This helps you land properly and away from other players.

  - If you are undergoing muscle cramps, get off the field and take some rest. Playing through the pain may look brave, but later you would need to set yourself up for an extended time off the field.

Wrestling

Wrestling is a one-on-one duel where the stronger and quicker among the two emerges as a winner. During this game, injuries are likely. The most common sports injuries are sprains and strains. Shoulder separation or dislocation, kneecap dislocation, and prepatellar bursitis are some less common but serious injuries.

Safety Precautions To Follow

- Protect yourself with safety gear such as headgear, kneepads, shoes, mouthguard, and athletic support.

- Before you wrestle, take care of the following:

  - Get into good shape with a healthy diet and regular exercise. Do not lose weight the wrong way. This could leave you sluggish and weak on the wrestling floor. If you're planning to lose weight to compete in a specific weight category, lose your bulk systematically on a regular diet. Do not let anyone talk you into losing weight in a dangerous way.

  - Ensure the wrestling mat is cleaned with disinfectant before practice or match. Dirty mats are cause for infections such as impetigo and ringworm.

  - Before practice or competition, warm up with jumping jacks. Jog in place and do some dynamic stretching.

- While you are wrestling, take care of the following:

  - Master proper technique and learn to be quick with your moves with your opponent. This is as important as raw strength.

  - Avoid positions and holds that add stress on your elbows, shoulders, and knees. Be aware of dangerous positions that the referee will be on the lookout for to avoid fouls and disqualification.

  - If you are hurt or in pain ask for an injury time out. This will give you time to evaluate your position and you can decide if you want to continue or abandon a match for the sake of safety.

References

1. "Sports Safety Tips," Safe Kids Worldwide, 2016.
2. "Summer Sports Safety," New Jersey Division of Consumer Affairs, June 2, 2016.

3. "Preventing Children's Sports Injuries," Nemours, January 2015.

4. "Safety Tips: Football," Nemours, January 2014.

5. "Safety Tips: Baseball," Nemours, June 2014.

6. "Safety Tips: Basketball," Nemours, January 2014.

7. "Boxing Safety Tips," Life360 Inc., n.d.

8. Mackenzie B. "Track & Field Safety," BrianMac Sports Coach, 2000.

9. "Safety Tips: Soccer," Nemours, March 2014.

10. "Safety Tips: Volleyball," Nemours, June 2015.

11. "Safety Tips: Wrestling," Nemours, June 2015.

Chapter 25

Bike Safety

As you might expect, when a crash occurs between motor vehicle and a bike, it is the cyclist who is most likely to be injured. Bicyclists accounted for 2 percent of all traffic deaths and 2 percent of all crash-related injuries in 2014. Bicyclist deaths occurred most often between 6 p.m. and 9 p.m. (20%) and in urban areas (71%). The vast majority of bicyclists killed were male (88%). About one in five bicyclists (21%) killed in crashes had blood alcohol concentrations (BACs) of .08 grams per deciliter (g/dL) or higher, the illegal alcohol level in all States. A large percentage of crashes can be avoided if motorists and cyclists follow the rules of the road and watch out for each other.

Adolescents and young adults (15–19 years) and adults aged 40 years and older have the highest bicycle death rates.

Children (5–14 years), adolescents, and young adults (15–24 years) have the highest rates of nonfatal bicycle-related injuries, accounting for more than one-third of all bicycle-related injuries seen in U.S. emergency departments.

(Source: "Motor Vehicle Safety—Bicycle Safety," Centers for Disease Control and Prevention (CDC).)

Bicycle Safety

Americans are increasingly bicycling to commute, for exercise, or just for fun. By law, bicycles on the roadway are vehicles with the same rights and responsibilities as motorized

About This Chapter: This chapter includes text excerpted from "Road Safety—Bicyclists," National Highway Traffic Safety Administration (NHTSA), October 22, 2016.

vehicles. National Highway Traffic Safety Administration's (NHTSA) bicycle safety initiatives focus on encouraging safer choices on the part of bicyclists and drivers to help reduce deaths and injuries on our roads.

Helmet Fit

Every bike ride begins with putting on a helmet. But it's equally important that you ensure a proper fit so your helmet can best protect you.

Size can vary between manufacturers. Follow the steps to fit a helmet properly. It may take time to ensure a proper helmet fit, but your life is worth it. It's usually easier to look in the mirror or have someone else adjust the straps. For the most comprehensive list of helmet sizes according to manufacturers, go the Bicycle Helmet Safety Institute (BHSI) website at www.bhsi.org.

Avoid Crashes

Decreasing Risk Of Crashes

Ride your bike responsibly. All States require bicyclists on the roadway to follow the same rules and responsibilities as motorists.

There are two main types of crashes: the most common (falls), and the most serious (the ones with cars). Regardless of the reason for the crash, prevention is the name of the game; there are things you can do to decrease your risk of a crash.

Be Prepared Before Heading Out

- Ride a bike that fits you—if it's too big, it's harder to control the bike.

- Ride a bike that works—it really doesn't matter how well you ride if the brakes don't work.

- Wear equipment to protect you and make you more visible to others, like a bike helmet, bright clothing (during the day), reflective gear, and a white front light and red rear light and reflectors on your bike (at night, or when visibility is poor).

- Ride one per seat, with both hands on the handlebars, unless signaling a turn.

- Carry all items in a backpack or strapped to the back of the bike.

- Tuck and tie your shoelaces and pant legs so they don't get caught in your bike chain.

- Plan your route—if driving as a vehicle on the road, choose routes with less traffic and slower speeds. Your safest route may be away from traffic altogether, in a bike lane or on a bike path.

Drive Defensively—Focused And Alert

Be focused and alert to the road and all traffic around you; anticipate what others may do, before they do it. This is defensive driving—the quicker you notice a potential conflict, the quicker you can act to avoid a potential crash:

- Drive with the flow, in the same direction as traffic.

- Obey street signs, signals, and road markings, just like a car.

- Assume the other person doesn't see you; look ahead for hazards or situations to avoid that may cause you to fall, like toys, pebbles, potholes, grates, train tracks.

- No texting, listening to music or using anything that distracts you by taking your eyes and ears or your mind off the road and traffic.

Drive Predictably

By driving predictably, motorists get a sense of what you intend to do and can react to avoid a crash.

Drive where you are expected to be seen, travel in the same direction as traffic and signal and look over your shoulder before changing lane position or turning.

Avoid or minimize sidewalk riding. Cars don't expect to see moving traffic on a sidewalk and don't look for you when backing out of a driveway or turning. Sidewalks sometimes end unexpectedly, forcing the bicyclist into a road when a car isn't expecting to look for a bicyclist. If you must ride on the sidewalk remember to:

- Check your law to make sure sidewalk riding is legal;

- Watch for pedestrians;

- Pass pedestrians with care by first announcing "on your left" or "passing on your left" or use a bell;

- Ride in the same direction as traffic. This way, if the sidewalk ends, you are already riding with the flow of traffic. If crossing a street, motorists will look left, right, left for traffic. When you are to the driver's left, the driver is more likely to see you;

- Slow and look for traffic (left-right-left and behind) when crossing a street from a sidewalk; be prepared to stop and follow the pedestrian signals; and

- Slow down and look for cars backing out of driveways or turning.

Improve Your Riding Skills

No one learns to drive a vehicle safely without practice and experience; safely riding your bike in traffic requires the same preparation. Start by riding your bike in a safe environment away from traffic (a park, path, or empty parking lot).

Take an on-bike class through your school, recreation department, local bike shop or bike advocacy group. Confidence in traffic comes with learning how to navigate and communicate with other drivers, bicyclists, and pedestrians. Review and practice as a safe pedestrian or bicyclist is great preparation for safe riding.

Chapter 26

Skateboard Safety

Gear Up

Skateboards can be bought preassembled, or you can buy all of the pieces and put it together yourself. Preassembled boards are best for beginners, until you decide if skateboarding is really for you. If you are putting your own board together, you'll need a deck (the board itself), grip tape for the top of the deck so your feet don't slip, 2 trucks (the metal parts that are the axles of the wheels), 4 wheels, and 2 bearings per wheel (these keep the wheels spinning on the truck's axle). Before each time you ride, make sure your trucks are tightened and your wheels are spinning properly. Don't forget to wear a helmet, knee and elbow pads, and wrist guards. It's important that your helmet is approved by one of the groups who test helmets to see which ones are the best: the Snell B-95 standard is best for skateboarding helmets. Nonslippery shoes are a good idea too, so you can have better control of your board.

Play It Safe

Before you ride, make sure you give your board a safety check to make sure everything is put together right. Always wear all of your protective gear including a helmet, knee and elbow pads, and wrist guards. If you do tricks with your board, you may also want to wear gloves to protect your hands from the pavement. If you're just starting out, skate on a smooth, flat surface so you can practice keeping control of your board. And no matter how experienced you are—never hold on to the back of a moving vehicle! It's best to skate out of the way of traffic and other people (skate parks are great places to skate). But if you are skating in streets near your house,

About This Chapter: This chapter includes text excerpted from "BAM! Body And Mind—Skateboarding Activity Card," Centers for Disease Control and Prevention (CDC), May 9, 2015.

be aware of cars and people around you, and stay out of their way. Also, once the sun sets, it's a good idea to put up your board for the night, since skating in the dark can be dangerous.

Important Tips For Safer Riding

- Wear protective gear when riding—especially a helmet
- Stay clear of moving vehicles
- Inspect/adjust your board before you ride
- Ride during the day
- Inspect your riding terrain
- Never ride alone. Accidents happen
- Ride wisely
- Don't drink and ride

(Source: "Skateboarding Safety," U.S. Consumer Product Safety Commission (CPSC).)

How To Play

If you're just starting out, follow these steps to develop your skateboarding skills. Put one foot on the board, toward the front, with the other on the ground. Push off the ground with your foot and put it on the rear of the board while you glide. Push again when you slow down. If you start going too fast, step off the board with your back foot. To turn, shift your weight to your back foot so that the front truck lifts off the ground and then move your body in the direction you want to go—the board will go with you.

Speed Wobble

Speed wobble happens when a skateboard begins to shimmy from side to side unexpectedly. Within seconds, this can lead to a board rocking so violently that the rider is thrown to the ground before having a chance to react.

Ways to Reduce the Risk of Speed Wobble

- Ride forward and crouch on your board.
- Longer boards increase stability.
- Boards with wider hangers (wheels that are farther apart) give riders greater control.
- Keep trucks, wheels, nuts, and mounting screws tightened properly to improve stability at higher speeds.

(Source: "Skateboarding Safety," U.S. Consumer Product Safety Commission (CPSC).)

If you want to find half pipes, vert ramps, and skate courses near you to practice your moves, look for a nearby skate park, designed to give skateboarders a great ride.

There are several different styles of skateboarding:

- Street skating is skateboarding on streets, curbs, benches and handrails—anything involving common street objects. Street skating is best left to the pros though—it's very dangerous.

- Downhill skating is racing down big hills, usually on a longer skateboard called a longboard.

- Freestyle skating is more artistic, involving a series of tricks and stunts.

- Vert skating is skateboarding on mini-ramps and half pipes, which are U-shaped ramps.

Chapter 27

Football Safety

Gear Up

Always wear a helmet with a face mask and jaw pads, and a mouthpiece to protect against those hard hits. Because football is a contact sport, there are many different pieces of gear you should wear to protect different areas of your body. For upper body protection, you should wear a neck roll to prevent whiplash, shoulder pads, rib pads, arm pads and elbow pads. For leg protection, you should wear hip pads, tailbone pads, thigh pads, and knee pads. Most leagues require all this, but it's a good idea to protect yourself even in backyard games.

Play It Safe

Be sure to stretch and warm up before every practice and game and always wear your protective gear. To avoid getting hurt, learn from your coaches how to block and tackle correctly. Don't tackle with the top of your head or helmet—not only is it illegal, but it can cause injury to both players. If you play in an organized league, there are lots of rules—and they are there for a reason—to keep you safe. If you break these rules, you risk not only getting hurt, or hurting someone else, but your team will be penalized. If you're playing in the backyard with your friends, stay safe by sticking to touch or flag football, and only play with kids who are around your age and size.

About This Chapter: Text beginning with the heading "Gear Up" is excerpted from "BAM! Body And Mind—Football Activity Card," Centers for Disease Control and Prevention (CDC), May 9, 2015; Text beginning with the heading "Football Helmet Safety: Start With The Right Size" is excerpted from "Get A Heads Up On Football Helmet Safety," Centers for Disease Control and Prevention (CDC), July 14, 2013. Reviewed July 2017.

How To Play

There are lots of skills needed to play football from throwing and catching the ball to blocking and tackling the other players. There's even a national Punt, Pass, and Kick contest devoted just to the main skills you need. League teams are a great way to learn all the rules and strategies of football. Pop Warner is the most popular youth football league, but there are many others nationwide.

Throwing the ball. Grip the ball by placing each of your fingers between each lace of the ball. Bring your throwing arm back with your elbow bent. Extend your free arm (the one without the ball) in front of you and point to your target. Snap your throwing arm forward, releasing the ball, and follow through with your shoulders and hips. When you are finished, your throwing arm should be pointing toward your target with your palm facing the ground.

Catching the ball. Hold your arms out with your elbows slightly bent in front of your chest. Bring your hands together, touching the thumbs and index fingers to make a triangle with your fingers. Catch the nose of the ball in the triangle, and use your chest to help trap the ball. Bring your arms in around the ball and hold it tight against you.

Punting the ball. Place your feet shoulder-width apart with your kicking foot slightly in front. Slightly bend your knees and bend your body forward a little. Hold the ball out in front of you with the laces facing upward. Take two steps forward, beginning with your kicking foot and drop the ball toward your kicking foot. Kick the ball hard with the top of your foot and follow through with your leg as high as you can.

Football Helmet Safety: Start With The Right Size

Bring The Athlete

Bring your athlete with you when buying a new helmet to make sure that you can check for a good fit.

Head Size

To find out the size of your athlete's head, wrap a soft tape measure around the athlete's head, just above their eyebrows and ears. Make sure the tape measure stays level from front to back. (If you don't have a soft tape measure, you can use a string and then measure it against a ruler.)

Sizes Will Vary

Helmet sizes often will vary from brand-to-brand and with different models. Each helmet will fit differently, so it is important to check out the manufacturer's website for the helmet brand's fit instructions and sizing charts, as well as to find out what helmet size fits your athlete's head size.

Get A Good Fit

General Fit

A football helmet should feel snug with no spaces between the pads and the athlete's head. The helmet should not slide on the head with the chin strap in place. If the helmet can be removed while the chin strap is in place, then the fit is too loose. Some helmets have a unique fitting system or use an air bladder system that requires inflation with a special needle to avoid puncturing the air bladders.

Ask

Ask your athlete how the helmet feels on their head. While it needs to have a snug fit, a helmet that is too tight can cause headaches.

Hairstyle

Your athlete should try on the helmet with the hairstyle he will wear while at practices and games. Helmet fit can change if your athlete's hairstyle changes. For example, a long-haired athlete who gets a very short haircut may need to adjust the fit of the helmet.

Coverage

A football helmet should not sit too high or low on their head. To check, make sure ear holes line up with athlete's ears, and helmet pad covers athlete's head from middle of his forehead to back of his head.

Vision

Make sure you can see your athlete's eyes and that he can see straight forward and side-to-side.

Chin Straps

The chin strap should be centered under the athlete's chin and fit snugly. Tell your athlete to open their mouth wide…big yawn! The helmet should pull down on their head. If not, the chin strap needs to be tighter. Once the chin strap is fastened, the helmet should not move in any direction, back-to-front or side-to-side.

Take Care Of The Helmet

Check For Damage

DO NOT allow your athlete to use a cracked or broken helmet or a helmet that is missing any padding or parts. For air bladder-equipped helmets, make sure to check for proper inflation. DO NOT alter, remove or replace padding or internal parts unless supervised by a trained equipment manager. Check for missing or loose parts and padding before the season and regularly during the season.

Cleaning

Clean the helmet often inside and out with warm water and mild detergent. DO NOT soak any part of the helmet, put it close to high heat, or use strong cleaners.

Protect

DO NOT let anyone sit or lean on the helmet.

Storage

Do not store a football helmet in a car. The helmet should be stored in a room that does not get too hot or too cold and where the helmet is away from direct sunlight.

Decoration

DO NOT decorate (paint or put stickers on) the helmet without checking with the helmet manufacturer, as this may affect the safety of the helmet. This information may also be found on the instructions label or on the manufacturer's website.

Look For A Football Helmet With Labels That

- Have the date of manufacture. This information will be helpful in case the helmet is recalled; and

- Say National Operating Committee on Standards for Athletic Equipment (NOCSAE®) certified. That label means that the helmet has been tested for safety and meets safety standards.

If the helmet is not new, you should also look for a label that includes the date the helmet was expertly repaired and approved for use (reconditioned/recertified). Helmets that have been properly reconditioned and recertified will have a label with the date of recertification and the name of the reconditioning company.

Know When To Replace A Football Helmet

Reconditioning

Reconditioning involves having an expert inspect and repair a used helmet by: fixing cracks or damage, replacing missing parts, testing it for safety, and recertifying it for use. Helmets should be reconditioned regularly by a licensed National Athletic Equipment Reconditioner Association (NAERA)-member. DO NOT allow your athlete to use a used helmet that is not approved/recertified for use by a NAERA reconditioner.

10 And Out

Football helmets should be replaced no later than 10 years from the date of manufacture. Many helmets will need to be replaced sooner, depending upon wear and tear.

Chapter 28

Water Sports Safety

Every day, about ten people die from unintentional drowning. Of these, two are children aged 14 or younger. Drowning ranks fifth among the leading causes of unintentional injury death in the United States.

How Big Is The Problem?

- From 2005–2014, there were an average of 3,536 fatal unintentional drownings (non-boating related) annually in the United States—about ten deaths per day. An additional 332 people died each year from drowning in boating-related incidents.

- About one in five people who die from drowning are children 14 and younger. For every child who dies from drowning, another five receive emergency department care for non-fatal submersion injuries.

- More than 50 percent of drowning victims treated in emergency departments (EDs) require hospitalization or transfer for further care (compared with a hospitalization rate of about 6 percent for all unintentional injuries). These nonfatal drowning injuries can cause severe brain damage that may result in long-term disabilities such as memory problems, learning disabilities, and permanent loss of basic functioning (e.g., permanent vegetative state).

About This Chapter: Text in this chapter begins with excerpts from "Recreational Safety—Unintentional Drowning: Get The Facts," Centers for Disease Control and Prevention (CDC), May 2, 2016; Text under the heading "Recreational Water Illnesses (RWI)" is excerpted from "Healthy Swimming—Recreational Water Illnesses," Centers for Disease Control and Prevention (CDC), January 25, 2017.

Risk Factors

Who Is Most At Risk?

- **Males:** Nearly 80 percent of people who die from drowning are male.

- **Children:** Children ages 1 to 4 have the highest drowning rates. In 2014, among children 1 to 4 years old who died from an unintentional injury, one-third died from drowning. Among children ages 1 to 4, most drownings occur in home swimming pools. Drowning is responsible for more deaths among children 1–4 than any other cause except congenital anomalies (birth defects). Among those 1–14, fatal drowning remains the second-leading cause of unintentional injury-related death behind motor vehicle crashes.

- **Minorities:** Between 1999–2010, the fatal unintentional drowning rate for African Americans was significantly higher than that of whites across all ages. The disparity is widest among children 5–18 years old. The disparity is most pronounced in swimming pools; African American children 5–19 drown in swimming pools at rates 5.5 times higher than those of whites. This disparity is greatest among those 11–12 years where African Americans drown in swimming pools at rates 10 times those of whites.

Factors such as access to swimming pools, the desire or lack of desire to learn how to swim, and choosing water-related recreational activities may contribute to the racial differences in drowning rates. Available rates are based on population, not on participation. If rates could be determined by actual participation in water-related activities, the disparity in minorities' drowning rates compared to whites would be much greater.

What Factors Influence Drowning Risk?

The main factors that affect drowning risk are lack of swimming ability, lack of barriers to prevent unsupervised water access, lack of close supervision while swimming, location, failure to wear life jackets, alcohol use, and seizure disorders.

- **Lack of Swimming Ability:** Many adults and children report that they can't swim. Research has shown that participation in formal swimming lessons can reduce the risk of drowning among children aged 1 to 4 years.

- **Lack of Barriers:** Barriers, such as pool fencing, prevent young children from gaining access to the pool area without caregivers' awareness. A four-sided isolation fence (separating the pool area from the house and yard) reduces a child's risk of drowning 83 percent compared to three-sided property-line fencing.

- **Lack of Close Supervision:** Drowning can happen quickly and quietly anywhere there is water (such as bathtubs, swimming pools, buckets), and even in the presence of lifeguards.

- **Location:** People of different ages drown in different locations. For example, most children ages 1–4 drown in home swimming pools. The percentage of drownings in natural water settings, including lakes, rivers and oceans, increases with age. More than half of fatal and nonfatal drownings among those 15 years and older (57% and 57% respectively) occurred in natural water settings.

- **Failure to Wear Life Jackets:** In 2010, the U.S. Coast Guard (USCG) received reports for 4,604 boating incidents; 3,153 boaters were reported injured, and 672 died. Most (72%) boating deaths that occurred during 2010 were caused by drowning, with 88 percent of victims not wearing life jackets.

- **Alcohol Use:** Among adolescents and adults, alcohol use is involved in up to 70 percent of deaths associated with water recreation, almost a quarter of ED visits for drowning, and about one in five reported boating deaths. Alcohol influences balance, coordination, and judgment, and its effects are heightened by sun exposure and heat.

- **Seizure Disorders:** For persons with seizure disorders, drowning is the most common cause of unintentional injury death, with the bathtub as the site of highest drowning risk.

Prevention

What Has Research Found?

- **Swimming skills help.** Taking part in in formal swimming lessons reduces the risk of drowning among children aged 1 to 4 years. However, many people don't have basic swimming skills. A Centers for Disease Control and Prevention (CDC) study about self-reported swimming ability found that:

  - Younger adults reported greater swimming ability than older adults.

  - Self-reported ability increased with level of education.

  - Among racial groups, African Americans reported the most limited swimming ability.

  - Men of all ages, races, and educational levels consistently reported greater swimming ability than women.

- **Seconds count—learn Cardiopulmonary Resuscitation (CPR).** CPR performed by bystanders has been shown to save lives and improve outcomes in drowning victims. The more quickly CPR is started, the better the chance of improved outcomes.

- **Life jackets can reduce risk.** Potentially, half of all boating deaths might be prevented with the use of life jackets.

Tips To Help You Stay Safe In The Water

- **Supervise When in or Around Water.** Designate a responsible adult to watch young children while in the bath and all children swimming or playing in or around water. Supervisors of preschool children should provide "touch supervision," be close enough to reach the child at all times. Because drowning occurs quickly and quietly, adults should not be involved in any other distracting activity (such as reading, playing cards, talking on the phone, or mowing the lawn) while supervising children, even if lifeguards are present.

- **Use the Buddy System.** Always swim with a buddy. Select swimming sites that have lifeguards when possible.

- **Seizure Disorder Safety.** If you or a family member has a seizure disorder, provide one-on-one supervision around water, including swimming pools. Consider taking showers rather than using a bathtub for bathing. Wear life jackets when boating.

- **Learn to Swim.** Formal swimming lessons can protect young children from drowning. However, even when children have had formal swimming lessons, constant, careful supervision when children are in the water, and barriers, such as pool fencing to prevent unsupervised access, are still important.

- **Learn Cardiopulmonary Resuscitation (CPR).** In the time it takes for paramedics to arrive, your CPR skills could save someone's life.

- **Air-Filled or Foam Toys are not safety devices.** Don't use air-filled or foam toys, such as "water wings," "noodles," or inner-tubes, instead of life jackets. These toys are not life jackets and are not designed to keep swimmers safe.

- **Avoid Alcohol.** Avoid drinking alcohol before or during swimming, boating, or water skiing. Do not drink alcohol while supervising children.

- **Don't let swimmers hyperventilate before swimming underwater or try to hold their breath for long periods of time.** This can cause them to pass out (sometimes called "hypoxic blackout" or "shallow water blackout") and drown.

- **Know how to prevent recreational water illnesses.**

- **Know the local weather conditions and forecast before swimming or boating.** Strong winds and thunderstorms with lightning strikes are dangerous.

Safety While Boating

- Wear your personal floatation device (PFD) and make sure that your passengers wear theirs, too!
- If operating a houseboat, be careful of carbon monoxide buildup around the boat. Also use caution around the electrical connections to the boat slip or dock.
- Obey the posted speedlimits and wake warnings.
- Do not operate your watercraft on unauthorized waterways.
- Never consume alcohol while operating a watercraft.
- Bring along extra safety items such as water, flashlights, maps, and a cellphone or radio.

(Source: "Water Sports," Recreation.gov.)

If You Have A Swimming Pool At Home

- **Install Four-Sided Fencing.** Install a four-sided pool fence that completely separates the pool area from the house and yard. The fence should be at least 4 feet high. Use self-closing and self-latching gates that open outward with latches that are out of reach of children. Also, consider additional barriers such as automatic door locks and alarms to prevent access or alert you if someone enters the pool area.

- **Clear the Pool and Deck of Toys.** Remove floats, balls and other toys from the pool and surrounding area immediately after use so children are not tempted to enter the pool area unsupervised.

If You Are In And Around Natural Water Settings

- **Use U.S. Coast Guard approved life jackets.** This is important regardless of the distance to be traveled, the size of the boat, or the swimming ability of boaters; life jackets can reduce risk for weaker swimmers too.

- **Know the meaning of and obey warnings represented by colored beach flags.** These may vary from one beach to another.

- **Watch for dangerous waves and signs of rip currents.** Some examples are water that is discolored and choppy, foamy, or filled with debris and moving in a channel away from shore.

157

- **If you are caught in a rip current, swim parallel to shore.** Once free of the current, swim diagonally toward shore.

Recreational Water Illnesses (RWIs)

What Are RWIs?

Recreational water illnesses (RWIs) are caused by germs spread by swallowing, breathing in mists or aerosols of, or having contact with contaminated water in swimming pools, hot tubs, water parks, water play areas, interactive fountains, lakes, rivers, or oceans. RWIs can also be caused by chemicals in the water or chemicals that evaporate from the water and cause indoor air quality problems. RWIs can be a wide variety of infections, including gastrointestinal, skin, ear, respiratory, eye, neurologic and wound infections. The most commonly reported RWI is diarrhea. Diarrheal illnesses can be caused by germs such as Crypto (short for *Cryptosporidium*), *Giardia, Shigella, norovirus,* and *E. coli O157:H7.*

Why Should We Be Interested In RWIs?

Contrary to popular belief, chlorine does not kill all germs instantly. There are germs today that are very tolerant to chlorine and were not known to cause human disease until recently. Once these germs get in the pool, it can take anywhere from minutes to days for chlorine to kill them. Swallowing just a little water that contains these germs can make you sick.

In the past two decades, there has been a substantial increase in the number of RWI outbreaks associated with swimming. Crypto, which can stay alive for days even in well-maintained pools, has become the leading cause of swimming pool-related outbreaks of diarrheal illness.

Although Crypto is tolerant to chlorine, most germs are not. Keeping chlorine at recommended levels is essential to maintain a healthy pool. However, a study found that 1 in 8 public pool inspections resulted in pools being closed immediately due to serious code violations such as improper chlorine levels.

Where Are RWIs Found?

RWIs are caused by germs spread through contaminated water in swimming pools, water parks, water play areas, hot tubs, decorative water fountains, oceans, lakes, and rivers.

Swimming Pools, Water Parks, And Water Play Areas

The most common RWI is diarrhea. Swallowing even a small amount of water that has been contaminated with feces containing germs can cause diarrheal illness.

To ensure that most germs are killed, check chlorine or other disinfectant levels and pH regularly as part of good pool operation.

Hot Tubs

Skin infections like "hot tub rash" are a common RWI spread through hot tubs and spas. Respiratory illnesses are also associated with the use of improperly maintained hot tubs.

The high water temperatures in most hot tubs make it hard to maintain the disinfectant levels needed to kill germs. That's why it's important to check disinfectant levels in hot tubs even more regularly than in swimming pools.

The germs that cause "hot tub rash" can also be spread in pools that do not have proper disinfectant levels and in natural bodies of water such as oceans, lakes, or rivers.

Decorative Water Fountains

Not all decorative fountains are chlorinated or filtered. Therefore, when people, especially diaper-aged children, play in the water, they can contaminate the water with fecal matter. Swallowing this contaminated water can then cause diarrheal illness.

Oceans, Lakes, And Rivers

Oceans, lakes, and rivers can be contaminated with germs from sewage spills, animal waste, water runoff following rainfall, fecal incidents, and germs rinsed off the bottoms of swimmers. It is important to avoid swallowing the water because natural recreational water is not disinfected. Avoid swimming after rainfalls or in areas identified as unsafe by health departments.

How Are RWIs Spread?

Diarrheal Illnesses

Swallowing water that has been contaminated with feces containing germs can cause diarrheal illness.

Swimmers share the water—and the germs in it—with every person who enters the pool. On average, people have about 0.14 grams of feces on their bottoms 1 which, when rinsed off, can contaminate recreational water. In addition, when someone is ill with diarrhea, their stool can contain millions of germs. This means that just one person with diarrhea can easily contaminate the water in a large pool or water park. Swallowing even a small amount of recreational water that has been contaminated with feces containing germs can make you sick. Remember, chlorine does not kill germs instantly, and some germs, such as Cryptosporidium (or "Crypto"), are extremely chlorine tolerant.

In addition, lakes, rivers, and the ocean can be contaminated with germs from sewage spills, animal waste, and water runoff following rainfall. Some common germs can also live for long periods of time in salt water.

Other RWIs

Many other RWIs (skin, ear, eye, respiratory, neurologic, wound, and other infections) are caused by germs that live naturally in the environment (for example, in water and soil). If disinfectant levels in pools or hot tubs are not maintained at the appropriate levels, these germs can multiply and cause illness when swimmers breathe in mists or aerosols of or have contact with the contaminated water.

Why Doesn't Chlorine Kill RWI Germs?

Chlorine (in swimming pools and hot tubs) kills the germs that cause RWIs, but the time it takes to kill each germ varies.

In pools and hot tubs with the correct pH and disinfectant levels, chlorine will kill most germs that cause RWIs in less than an hour. However, chlorine takes longer to kill some germs, such as Crypto (short for Cryptosporidium). Crypto can survive for days even in a properly disinfected pool. This is why it is so important for swimmers to keep germs out of the water in the first place.

Who Is Most Likely To Get Ill From An RWI?

Children, pregnant women, and people with weakened immune systems (for example, people living with AIDS, individuals who have received an organ transplant, or people receiving certain types of chemotherapy) can suffer from more severe illness if infected. People with weakened immune systems should be aware that recreational water might be contaminated with human or animal feces containing Crypto (short for *Cryptosporidium*). Crypto can cause a life-threatening infection in persons with weakened immune systems.

People with a weakened immune system should consult their healthcare provider before participating in activities that place them at risk for illness.

How Can We Prevent RWIs?

There are a few easy and effective healthy swimming steps all swimmers can take each time we swim to help protect ourselves, our families, and our friends from RWIs.

What Are The Top Causes Of All RWI Outbreaks?

1. Cryptosporidium

2. Pseudomonas

3. Shigella

4. Legionella

5. Norovirus

6. *E. coli*

7. Giardia

8. Disinfection agents and their byproducts (chlorine, bromine, hydrochloric acid)

9. Avian schistosomes

10. Leptospira

Chapter 29

Winter Sports Safety

Concussion In Winter Sports

Each winter, hundreds of thousands of young athletes head out to ice and ski slopes to enjoy, practice, and compete in various winter sports. There's no doubt that these sports are a great way for kids and teens to stay healthy, as well as learn important leadership and team-building skills. But there are risks to pushing the limits of speed, strength, and endurance. And athletes who push the limits sometimes don't recognize their own *limitations*—especially when they've had a concussion.

A concussion is a type of traumatic brain injury—or TBI—caused by a bump, blow, or jolt to the head or by a hit to the body that causes the head and brain to move rapidly back and forth. This sudden movement can cause the brain to bounce around or twist in the skull, stretching and damaging the brain cells and creating chemical changes in the brain.

While most athletes with a concussion recover quickly and fully, some will have symptoms that last for days or even weeks. A more serious concussion can last for months or longer.

About This Chapter: Text under the heading "Concussion In Winter Sports" is excerpted from "Concussion In Winter Sports," Centers for Disease Control and Prevention (CDC), December 24, 2012. Reviewed July 2017; Text under the heading "Head And Neck Injuries In Winter Sports" is excerpted from "Head And Neck Injuries In Winter Sports," Office of Disease Prevention and Health Promotion (ODPHP), U.S. Department of Health and Human Services (HHS), January 20, 2016; Text under the heading "Frostbite" is excerpted from "Natural Disasters and Severe Weather—Frostbite," Centers for Disease Control and Prevention (CDC), December 20, 2016; Text under the heading "Hypothermia" is excerpted from "Natural Disasters and Severe Weather—Hypothermia," Centers for Disease Control and Prevention (CDC), December 20, 2016; Text under the heading "Snowboard Helmet Safety" is excerpted from "Get A Heads Up On Snowboard Helmet Safety," Centers for Disease Control and Prevention (CDC), July 14, 2013. Reviewed July 2017.

That's why Centers for Disease Control and Prevention (CDC) and the National Football League (NFL) teamed up with USA Hockey, the U.S. Ski and Snowboarding Association (USSA), and 12 other national governing bodies for sports to develop a poster for young athletes. This poster lets athletes know that all concussions are serious and emphasizes the importance of reporting their injury. It also provides athletes with a list of concussion signs, symptoms, and steps they should take if they think they have a concussion.

The poster was created through CDC's "Heads Up" educational campaign that includes resources for high school and youth sports coaches, school professionals, and healthcare professionals. These initiatives include materials and information to help identify concussions and immediate steps to take when one is suspected.

Prevention And Preparation: On And Off The Ice And Ski Slopes

Insist that safety comes first. No one technique or safety equipment is 100 percent effective in preventing concussion, but there are things you can do to help minimize the risks for concussion and other injuries.

For example, to help prevent injuries:

- Make sure to wear approved and properly-fitted protective equipment. Such equipment should be well-maintained and be worn consistently and correctly.

- Enforce no hits to the head or other types of dangerous play in hockey and other sports.

- Practice safe playing techniques and encourage athletes to follow the rules of play.

Learn about concussion. Before strapping on your skates, skis or snowboard, learn concussion symptoms and dangers signs, and their potential long-term consequences.

Order and display the concussion poster. CDC and the NFL encourage parents, coaches, and school professionals to display this poster in team locker rooms, competition and tournament sites, gymnasiums, ice rinks, and schools nationwide.

Head And Neck Injuries In Winter Sports

With the growth of the X Games, winter "extreme" sports like freestyle skiing and snowboarding are as popular as ever. These sports send athletes far into the air and down the slopes and ramps at tremendous speeds. Injuries, especially concussions and other traumatic brain injuries (TBI), unfortunately can occur.

Knowing just how common these injuries are in winter sports can help us take steps to prevent some of these brain injuries.

Extreme Sports Injuries To The Head And Neck

A study published in the *Orthopaedic Journal of Sports Medicine (OJSM)* looked at the incidence of head and neck injuries in seven extreme sports—snowboarding, snow skiing, snowmobiling, surfing, skateboarding, mountain biking, and motocross. The study is helpful to provide injury data, as these sports often lack the ability for organizing bodies to track participants. Plus this study allows us to compare rates of concussions in winter sports like skiing and snowboarding to the risks in warm-weather activities.

The study's findings are summarized below:

- Skateboarding, snowboarding, skiing and motocross had the highest number of head and neck injuries. Mountain biking, snowmobiling, and surfing had the lowest numbers.

- Snowboarding had the most concussions. In fact, about 30 percent of concussions in extreme sports occurred in snowboarding. Snow skiing was associated with about 25 percent of concussions.

- Skateboarding and motocross had the most severe head and neck injuries, like skull fractures and cervical spine fractures.

Tips To Prevent Head Injuries In Winter Sports

While the data might seem frightening, there are some steps that might decrease your chance of suffering traumatic brain injuries in winter sports:

- Wear a helmet. Helmets are critical in extreme winter sports like skiing and snowboarding, which account for a significant number of concussions.

- Do everything possible to optimize the conditions where you are performing these activities. Stay within the marked boundaries on the slopes and watch out for obstacles and hazardous conditions.

- Try to participate in these activities in places where medical care is not far away. Professional competitions have doctors and emergency medical services, but many people perform these activities in remote locations. Seek medical attention if there is any question that you might have suffered a traumatic brain injury, no matter how minor it might seem.

Frostbite

What Is Frostbite?

Frostbite is a serious condition that's caused by exposure to extremely cold temperatures. Stay safe this winter by learning more about frostbite, including who is most at risk, signs and symptoms, and what to do if someone develops frostbite.

Frostbite is a bodily injury caused by freezing that results in loss of feeling and color in affected areas. It most often affects the nose, ears, cheeks, chin, fingers, or toes. Frostbite can permanently damage the body, and severe cases can lead to amputation.

Recognizing Frostbite

At the first signs of redness or pain in any skin area, get out of the cold or protect any exposed skin—frostbite may be beginning. Any of the following signs may indicate frostbite:

- a white or grayish-yellow skin area

- skin that feels unusually firm or waxy

- numbness

A victim is often unaware of frostbite until someone else points it out because the frozen tissues are numb.

What To Do

If you detect symptoms of frostbite, seek medical care. First determine whether the victim also shows signs of hypothermia. Hypothermia is a more serious medical condition and requires emergency medical assistance.

If there is frostbite but no sign of hypothermia and immediate medical care is not available, proceed as follows:

- Get into a warm room as soon as possible.

- Unless absolutely necessary, do not walk on frostbitten feet or toes—this increases the damage.

- Immerse the affected area in warm—not hot—water (the temperature should be comfortable to the touch for unaffected parts of the body).

- Or, warm the affected area using body heat. For example, the heat of an armpit can be used to warm frostbitten fingers.

- Do not rub the frostbitten area with snow or massage it at all. This can cause more damage.

- Don't use a heating pad, heat lamp, or the heat of a stove, fireplace, or radiator for warming. Affected areas are numb and can be easily burned.

These procedures are not substitutes for proper medical care. Hypothermia is a medical emergency and frostbite should be evaluated by a healthcare provider.

Be Prepared

Taking a first aid and emergency resuscitation (CPR) course is a good way to prepare for cold-weather health problems. Knowing what to do is an important part of protecting your health and the health of others.

Taking preventive action is your best defense against having to deal with extreme cold-weather conditions. By preparing your home and car in advance for winter emergencies, and by observing safety precautions during times of extremely cold weather, you can reduce the risk of weather-related health problems.

Hypothermia

What Is Hypothermia?

Hypothermia, or abnormally low body temperature, is a dangerous condition that can occur when a person is exposed to extremely cold temperatures. Stay safe this winter by learning more about hypothermia, including who is most at risk, signs and symptoms, and what to do if someone develops hypothermia.

Hypothermia is caused by prolonged exposures to very cold temperatures. When exposed to cold temperatures, your body begins to lose heat faster than it's produced. Lengthy exposures will eventually use up your body's stored energy, which leads to lower body temperature.

Body temperature that is too low affects the brain, making the victim unable to think clearly or move well. This makes hypothermia especially dangerous, because a person may not know that it's happening and won't be able to do anything about it. While hypothermia is most likely at very cold temperatures, it can occur even at cool temperatures (above 40°F) if a person becomes chilled from rain, sweat, or submersion in cold water.

Recognizing Hypothermia

- Shivering, exhaustion

- Confusion, fumbling hands
- Memory loss, slurred speech drowsiness
- Bright red, cold skin
- Very low energy

Take Action

If you notice any of these signs, take the person's temperature. If it is below 95° F, the situation is an emergency—get medical attention immediately.

If medical care is not available, begin warming the person, as follows:

- Get the victim into a warm room or shelter.
- If the victim has on any wet clothing, remove it.
- Warm the center of the body first—chest, neck, head, and groin—using an electric blanket, if available. You can also use skin-to-skin contact under loose, dry layers of blankets, clothing, towels, or sheets.
- Warm beverages can help increase body temperature, but do not give alcoholic beverages. Do not try to give beverages to an unconscious person.
- After body temperature has increased, keep the person dry and wrapped in a warm blanket, including the head and neck.
- Get medical attention as soon as possible.

A person with severe hypothermia may be unconscious and may not seem to have a pulse or to be breathing. In this case, handle the victim gently, and get emergency assistance immediately. Even if the victim appears dead, CPR should be provided. CPR should continue while the victim is being warmed, until the victim responds or medical aid becomes available. In some cases, hypothermia victims who appear to be dead can be successfully resuscitated.

Be Prepared

Taking a first aid and emergency resuscitation (CPR) course is a good way to prepare for cold-weather health problems. Knowing what to do is an important part of protecting your health and the health of others.

Taking preventive action is your best defense against having to deal with extreme cold-weather conditions. By preparing your home and car in advance for winter emergencies, and by observing safety precautions during times of extremely cold weather, you can reduce the risk of weather-related health problems.

Snowboard Helmet Safety

Start With The Right Size

Bring The Snowboarder

Children or teens can accompany when elders buy a new helmet for you to make sure that you can check for a good fit.

Head Size

Children or teens can find out the size of their head by wrapping a soft tape measure around his or her head, just above their eyebrows and ears. Make sure the tape measure stays level from front to back. (If you don't have a soft tape measure, you can use a string and then measure it against a ruler.)

Sizes Will Vary

Helmet sizes often will vary from brand-to-brand and with different models. Each helmet will fit differently, so it is important to check out the manufacturer's website for the helmet brand's fit instructions and sizing charts, as well as to find out what helmet size fits the child's or teen's head size.

Get A Good Fit

General Fit

A snowboard helmet should fit snugly all around, with no spaces between the foam or padding and the snowboarder's head.

Ask

Children or teens must be asked on how the helmet feels on their head. While it needs to have a snug fit, a helmet that is too tight can cause headaches.

Hairstyle

Children or teens should try on the helmet with the hairstyle he or she will wear while snowboarding. Helmet fit can change if the child's or teen's hairstyle changes. For example, a long-haired snowboarder who gets a very short haircut may need to adjust the fit of the helmet.

Coverage

A snowboard helmet should not sit too high or low on their head. To check, make sure the helmet sits low enough in the front to protect the snowboarder's forehead, about 1 inch above the eyebrows, and the back of the helmet does not touch the top of the snowboarder's neck.

Adjustments

Some snowboard helmets have removable padding that can be adjusted to get a good fit.

Goggles

Children or teens should try on the helmet with the goggles they will wear on the slopes. The helmet should fit snugly on top of the goggles, with no space between the helmet and the top of the goggles. However, the helmet should not sit so low on the snowboarder's head that it pushes down on the goggles.

Vision

Make sure that the snowboarder can see straight forward and side-to-side.

Chin Straps

The chin strap should be centered under the snowboarder's chin and fit snugly, so that no more than one or two fingers fit between the chin and the strap. Children or teens should to open their mouth wide…big yawn! The helmet should pull down on their head. If not, the chin strap needs to be tighter. Once the chin strap is fastened, the helmet should not move in any direction, back-to-front or side-to-side.

Take Care Of The Helmet

Check For Damage

DO NOT allow your snowboarder to use a cracked or broken helmet or a helmet that is missing any padding or parts.

Cleaning

Clean the helmet often inside and out with warm water and mild detergent. DO NOT soak any part of the helmet, put it close to high heat, or use strong cleaners.

Protect

DO NOT let anyone sit or lean on the helmet.

Storage

Do not store a snowboard helmet in a car. The helmet should be stored in a room that does not get too hot or too cold and where the helmet is away from direct sunlight.

Decoration

DO NOT decorate (paint or put stickers on) the helmet without checking with the helmet manufacturer, as this may affect the safety of the helmet. This information may also be found on the instructions label or on the manufacturer's website.

Look For A Snowboard Helmet With Labels That

- Have the date of manufacture. This information will be helpful in case the helmet is recalled; and

- Say ASTM certified. That label means that the helmet has been tested for safety and meets safety standards.

When To Replace A Snowboarder's Helmet

Snowboard helmets are designed to withstand more than one very minor hit. However, a snowboard helmet MUST be replaced if it has been involved in a serious crash or is damaged.

Multi-Use Helmets

Some helmet companies have created multi-use helmets for biking, skateboarding, and other activities. Multi-use helmets are designed to withstand multiple very minor hits; however, a multi-use helmet MUST be replaced if it has been involved in a serious crash or is damaged. Before the child or teen uses a multi-use helmet for snowboarding, make sure the helmet has an ASTM label certifying it for snowboarding.

Tips For Winter Sports Safety

Be responsible when skiing, snowmobiling, and snowboarding with these quick tips:

- Low snow, don't go. Avoid areas with inadequate snow cover. Traveling in these conditions can damage plants and soils just below the snow's surface.
- Travel only in areas designated for your type of winter travel.

- Avoid traveling in potential avalanche areas. use terrain to your advantage, avoiding steep slopes, cornices, and gullies or depressions, periodically check for clues to an unstable snowpack. Remember, one person at a time on slopes. An avalanche transceiver, shovel, and probe should be worn on your body at all times in an avalanche terrain.
- Respect established ski tracks. If traveling by foot or snowshoe don't damage existing ski tracks.
- If a person develops hypothermia, warm the person up by rubbing them vigorously and getting them into dry clothes. Give them warm nonalcoholic liquids.
- If you must have a fire, use a fire pan.
- Dispose of all sanitary waste properly by backing it out or bury it in a shallow hole in the snow.

(Source: "Winter Sports Safety," U.S. Department of Agriculture (USDA).)

Chapter 30

Preventing Sports Injuries

Although sports participation provides numerous physical and social benefits, it also has a downside: the risk of sports-related injuries. According to the Centers for Disease Control and Prevention (CDC), more than 2.6 million children 0–19 years old are treated in the emergency department each year for sports and recreation-related injuries.

These injuries are by far the most common cause of musculoskeletal injuries in children treated in emergency departments. They are also the single most common cause of injury-related primary care office visits.

The Most Common Musculoskeletal Sports-Related Injuries In Kids

Although sports injuries can range from scrapes and bruises to serious brain and spinal cord injuries, most fall somewhere between the two extremes. Here are some of the more common types of injuries.

Sprains And Strains

A sprain is an injury to a ligament, one of the bands of tough, fibrous tissue that connects two or more bones at a joint and prevents excessive movement of the joint. An ankle sprain is the most common athletic injury.

About This Chapter: This chapter includes text excerpted from "Preventing Musculoskeletal Sports Injuries In Youth: A Guide For Parents," National Institute of Arthritis and Musculoskeletal and Skin Diseases (NIAMS), September 2016.

A strain is an injury to either a muscle or a tendon. A muscle is a tissue composed of bundles of specialized cells that, when stimulated by nerve messages, contract and produce movement. A tendon is a tough, fibrous cord of tissue that connects muscle to bone. Muscles in any part of the body can be injured.

Growth Plate Injuries

In some sports accidents and injuries, the growth plate may be injured. The growth plate is the area of developing tissues at the end of the long bones in growing children and adolescents. When growth is complete, sometime during adolescence, the growth plate is replaced by solid bone. The long bones in the body include:

- the long bones of the hand and fingers (metacarpals and phalanges)

- both bones of the forearm (radius and ulna)

- the bone of the upper leg (femur)

- the lower leg bones (tibia and fibula)

- the foot bones (metatarsals and phalanges).

If any of these areas becomes injured, it's important to seek professional help from an orthopaedic surgeon, a doctor who specializes in bone injuries.

Repetitive Motion Injuries

Painful injuries such as stress fractures (a hairline fracture of the bone that has been subjected to repeated stress) and tendinitis (inflammation of a tendon) can occur from overuse of muscles and tendons. Some of these injuries don't always show up on X-rays, but they do cause pain and discomfort. The injured area usually responds to rest, ice, compression, and elevation (RICE). Other treatments can include crutches, cast immobilization, and physical therapy.

Preventing And Treating Musculoskeletal Injuries

Injuries can happen to any child who plays sports, but there are some things that can help prevent and treat injuries.

Prevention

- Children should be enrolled in organized sports through schools, community clubs, and recreation areas that are properly maintained. Any organized team activity should demonstrate a commitment to injury prevention. Coaches should be trained in first aid and cardiopulmonary resuscitation (CPR), and should have a plan for responding to emergencies. Coaches should be well versed in the proper use of equipment, and should enforce rules on equipment use.

- Organized sports programs may have adults on staff who are certified athletic trainers. These individuals are trained to prevent, recognize, and provide immediate care for athletic injuries.

- Make sure the child has—and consistently uses—proper gear for a particular sport. This may reduce the chances of being injured.

- Make warm-ups and cool-downs part of the child's routine before and after sports participation. Warm-up exercises make the body's tissues warmer and more flexible. Cool-down exercises loosen muscles that have tightened during exercise.

- Make sure the child has access to water or a sports drink while playing. Encourage him or her to drink frequently and stay properly hydrated. Remember to include sunscreen and a hat (when possible) to reduce the chance of sunburn, which is a type of injury to the skin. Sun protection may also decrease the chances of malignant melanoma—a potentially deadly skin cancer—or other skin cancers that can occur later in life.

- Learn and follow safety rules and suggestions for the child's particular sport. You'll find some more sport-specific safety suggestions below.

Key Prevention Tips

- **Gear up.** When children are active in sports and recreation, make sure they use the right protective gear for their activity, such as helmets, wrist guards, knee or elbow pads.

- **Use the right stuff.** Be sure that sports protective equipment is in good condition, fits appropriately and is worn correctly all the time—for example, avoid missing or broken buckles or compressed or worn padding. Poorly fitting equipment may be uncomfortable and may not offer the best protection.

- **Get an action plan in place.** Be sure the child's sports program or school has an action plan that includes information on how to teach athletes ways to lower their chances of getting a concussion and other injuries.

- **Pay attention to temperature.** Allow time for child athletes to gradually adjust to hot or humid environments to prevent heat-related injuries or illness. Parents and coaches should pay close attention to make sure that players are hydrated and appropriately dressed.

- **Be a good model.** Communicate positive safety messages and serve as a model of safe behavior, including wearing a helmet and following the rules.

(Source: "Child Safety And Injury Prevention," Centers for Disease Control and Prevention (CDC).)

Treatment

Treatment for sports-related injuries will vary by injury. But if the child suffers a soft tissue injury (such as a sprain or strain) or a bone injury, the best immediate treatment is easy to remember: RICE (rest, ice, compression, elevation) the injury. Get professional treatment if any injury is severe. A severe injury means having an obvious fracture or dislocation of a joint, prolonged swelling, or prolonged or severe pain.

Regular Exercise For Kids

It's important that kids continue some type of regular exercise after the injury heals. Exercise may reduce their chances of obesity, which has become more common in children. It may also reduce the risk of diabetes, a disease that can be associated with a lack of exercise and poor eating habits. Exercise also helps build social skills and provides a general sense of well-being. Sports participation is an important part of learning how to build team skills.

It's also important to match a child to the sport, and not push him or her too hard into an activity that he or she may not like or be capable of doing. Teach children to follow the rules and to play it safe when they get involved in sports, so they'll spend more time having fun in the game and be less likely to be sidelined with an injury. You should be mindful of the risks associated with different sports and take important measures to reduce the chance of injury.

Sport-Specific Safety Information

Here are some winning ways to help prevent an injury from occurring.

Basketball

- **Common injuries and locations:** Sprains, strains, bruises, fractures, scrapes, dislocations, cuts, injuries to teeth, ankles, and knees. (Injury rates are higher in girls, especially for the anterior cruciate ligament or ACL, the wide ligament that limits rotation and forward movement of the shin bone.)

- **Safest playing with:** Eye protection, elbow and knee pads, mouth guard, athletic supporters for males, proper shoes, water. If playing outdoors, wear sunscreen and, when possible, a hat.

- **Injury prevention:** Strength training (particularly knees and shoulders), aerobics (exercises that develop the strength and endurance of heart and lungs), warm-up exercises, proper coaching, use of safety equipment.

Track And Field

- **Common injuries:** Strains, sprains, scrapes from falls.

- **Safest playing with:** Proper shoes, athletic supporters for males, sunscreen, water.

- **Injury prevention:** Proper conditioning and coaching.

Football

- **Common injuries and locations:** Bruises, sprains, strains, pulled muscles, tears to soft tissues such as ligaments, broken bones, internal injuries (bruised or damaged organs), concussions, back injuries, sunburn. Knees and ankles are the most common injury sites.

- **Safest playing with:** Helmet, mouth guard, shoulder pads, athletic supporters for males, chest/rib pads, forearm, elbow, and thigh pads, shin guards, proper shoes, sunscreen, water.

- **Injury prevention:** Proper use of safety equipment, warm-up exercises, proper coaching techniques and conditioning.

Baseball And Softball

- **Common injuries:** Soft tissue strains, impact injuries that include fractures caused by sliding and being hit by a ball, sunburn.

- **Safest playing with:** Batting helmet; shin guards; elbow guards; athletic supporters for males; mouth guard; sunscreen; cleats; hat; detachable, "breakaway bases" rather than traditional, stationary ones.

- **Injury prevention:** Proper conditioning and warm-ups.

Soccer

- **Common injuries:** Bruises, cuts and scrapes, headaches, sunburn.

- **Safest playing with:** Shin guards, athletic supporters for males, cleats, sunscreen, water.

- **Injury prevention:** Aerobic conditioning and warm-ups, and—when age appropriate—proper training in "heading" (that is, using the head to strike or make a play with the ball).

Gymnastics

- **Common injuries:** Sprains and strains of soft tissues.

- **Safest playing with:** Athletic supporters for males, safety harness, joint supports (such as neoprene wraps), water.

- **Injury prevention:** Proper conditioning and warm-ups.

Treat Injuries With "RICE"

Rest: Reduce or stop using the injured area for at least 48 hours. If you have a leg injury, you may need to stay off of it completely.

Ice: Put an ice pack on the injured area for 20 minutes at a time, four to eight times per day. Use a cold pack, ice bag, or a plastic bag filled with crushed ice that has been wrapped in a towel.

Compression: Ask the child's doctor about elastics wraps, air casts, special boots, or splints that can be used to compress an injured ankle, knee, or wrist to reduce swelling.

Elevation: Keep the injured area elevated above the level of the heart to help decrease swelling. Use a pillow to help elevate an injured limb.

Part Three
Diagnosing And Treating Common Sports Injuries

Chapter 31

Understanding Sports Injuries

What Are Sports Injuries?

"Sports injuries" are injuries that happen when playing sports or exercising. Some are from accidents. Others can result from poor training practices or improper gear. Some people get injured when they are not in proper condition. Not warming up or stretching enough before you play or exercise can also lead to injuries.

The most common sports injuries are:

- Sprains and strains

- Knee injuries

- Swollen muscles

- Achilles tendon injuries

- Pain along the shin bone

- Fractures

- Dislocations

Sports-related injuries make up about 20 percent of all injury-related emergency department visits among children age 6 to 19.

(Source: "Common Sports Injuries: Incidence And Average Charges," Office of the Assistant Secretary for Planning and Evaluation (ASPE).)

About This Chapter: This chapter includes text excerpted from "Fast Facts About Sports Injuries," National Institute of Arthritis and Musculoskeletal and Skin Diseases (NIAMS), November 2014.

What's The Difference Between An Acute And A Chronic Injury?

There are two kinds of sports injuries: acute and chronic. Acute injuries occur suddenly when playing or exercising. Sprained ankles, strained backs, and fractured hands are acute injuries. Signs of an acute injury include:

- Sudden, severe pain

- Swelling

- Not being able to place weight on a leg, knee, ankle, or foot

- An arm, elbow, wrist, hand, or finger that is very tender

- Not being able to move a joint as normal

- Extreme leg or arm weakness

- A bone or joint that is visibly out of place

Chronic injuries happen after you play a sport or exercise for a long time. Signs of a chronic injury include:

- Pain when you play

- Pain when you exercise

- A dull ache when you rest

- Swelling

What Should I Do If I Get Injured?

Never try to "work through" the pain of a sports injury. Stop playing or exercising when you feel pain. Playing or exercising more only causes more harm. Some injuries should be seen by a doctor right away. Others you can treat yourself.

Call a doctor when:

- The injury causes severe pain, swelling, or numbness

- You can't put any weight on the area

- An old injury hurts or aches

- An old injury swells

- The joint doesn't feel normal or feels unstable.

If you don't have any of these signs, it may be safe to treat the injury at home. If the pain or other symptoms get worse, you should call your doctor. Use the RICE (Rest, Ice, Compression, and Elevation) method to relieve pain, reduce swelling, and speed healing. Follow these four steps right after the injury occurs and do so for at least 48 hours:

- **Rest.** Reduce your regular activities. If you've injured your foot, ankle, or knee, take weight off of it. A crutch can help. If your right foot or ankle is injured, use the crutch on the left side. If your left foot or ankle is injured, use the crutch on the right side.

- **Ice.** Put an ice pack to the injured area for 20 minutes, four to eight times a day. You can use a cold pack or ice bag. You can also use a plastic bag filled with crushed ice and wrapped in a towel. Take the ice off after 20 minutes to avoid cold injury.

- **Compression.** Put even pressure (compression) on the injured area to help reduce swelling. You can use an elastic wrap, special boot, air cast, or splint. Ask your doctor which one is best for your injury.

- **Elevation.** Put the injured area on a pillow, at a level above your heart, to help reduce swelling.

How Are Sports Injuries Treated?

Treatment often begins with the RICE method. Here are some other things your doctor may do to treat your sports injury.

- Nonsteroidal anti-inflammatory drugs (NSAIDs)

- Immobilization

- Surgery

- Rehabilitation (Exercise)

- Rest

- Other Therapies:

  - Mild electrical currents (electrostimulation)

  - Cold packs (cryotherapy)

  - Heat packs (thermotherapy)

  - Sound waves (ultrasound)

  - Massage

What Can People Do To Prevent Sports Injuries?

These tips can help you avoid sports injuries.

- Get a physical exam before you start playing sports.

- Do warm-up exercises before you play any sport.

- Be in proper condition to play the sport.

- Always stretch before you play or exercise.

- Don't overdo it.

- Don't bend your knees more than half way when doing knee bends.

- Don't twist your knees when you stretch. Keep your feet as flat as you can.

- When jumping, land with your knees bent.

- Wear shoes that fit properly, are stable, and absorb shock.

- Wear gear that protects, fits well, and is right for the sport.

- Know how to use athletic gear.

- Use the softest exercise surface you can find; don't run on asphalt or concrete.

- Run on flat surfaces.

- Don't play when you are very tired or in pain.

- Always cool down after you play.

- Follow the rules of the game.

Chapter 32

Overuse Injuries

Most sports-related injuries can be classified into one of two major types: acute macro-traumatic injuries, which are the result of a one-time inciting event, or chronic microtraumatic injuries, which occur over time and are often secondary to repetitive motions. Injuries in the latter group (also referred to as overuse or overload injuries) account for up to 50 percent of all sports-related injuries.

Pathophysiology

Generally, a tissue's response to any type of injury is inflammation. This inflammatory state is the initial phase of healing, lasting approximately 1–4 days. With overuse injuries, the inflammatory process becomes self-perpetuating, leading to the destruction of other surrounding tissues.

As the consequence of repetitive microtraumatic tensile overload, overuse injuries eventually lead to a disruption of the tissue's ability to repair itself. This results in the formation of scar tissue in place of the proper tissue matrix (i.e., bone, tendon, muscle, or ligament), which results in a decreased total tissue function for sport activity. With continued use, in the face of these tissue alterations, the individual may eventually experience symptoms in the form of pain, weakness, or diminished performance. It is, therefore, imperative that during treatment, this chronic inflammatory process be minimized to ensure adequate and proper tissue healing.

About This Chapter: This chapter includes text excerpted from "Overuse Syndrome Of The Upper Limb In People With Spinal Cord Injury," Rehabilitation Research & Development Service (RR&D), U.S. Department of Veterans Affairs (VA), December 27, 2016.

Overuse injuries most commonly affect the musculotendinous unit resulting in tendinitis, tenosynovitis, and/or muscle soreness. Other tissues that can be involved include: bursae (bursitis), bone (stress fractures), nerve (compression neuropathies), and cartilage (i.e., radiohumeral articular injury).

These overuse injuries can often have long-term consequences well into adulthood, including tendinitis, arthritis, and chronic pain.

(Source: "Aim To Stop Youth Sports Injuries," U.S. Department of Health and Human Services (HHS).)

Treatment And Rehabilitation

The treatment and rehabilitation of musculotendinous overuse injuries can be divided into four overlapping phases: (I) Inflammation and Pain Control; (II) Mobilization; (III) Strengthening; and (IV) Functional Restoration and Maintenance.

Phase I

Phase I is the initial stage of sport injury treatment. It incorporates measures that control both pain and inflammation while limiting further tissue damage. The PRICE (protection, relative rest, ice, compression, and elevation) protocol is commonly used and augmented with antiinflammatory medications. Phase I usually lasts from 1 to 2 weeks, but can persist for up to 6 weeks.

Protection in the form of immobilization (i.e., casting and splinting) is seldom required for extended periods of time with overuse injuries. Ice is used frequently during the first 24–48 hours postinjury to decrease both pain and edema, while compression bandages and elevation of the injured area are used to minimize swelling. A variety of heating modalities (i.e., heating pads, ultrasound, and whirlpool baths) can be utilized in the subacute postinjury period (1–2 days) if inflammation has been properly controlled. Heat acts to diminish painful muscle spasms and increase blood flow to the area, enhancing the healing process. Alternating ice and heat, known as contrast treatment, can also be used in the subacute phase.

Phase II

The mobilization phase of rehabilitation begins as soon as inflammation is controlled. The main goal of this phase is to regain and maintain normal range of motion of the injured body part. Prolonged immobilization of a joint will eventually lead to contracture formation and subsequent further deterioration in function.

Phase III

The strengthening phase of rehabilitation begins when from 80 to 85 percent painless range of motion is attained. It starts with isometric exercises and subsequently progresses to isotonic and isokinetic exercises as tolerated, making sure not to lose gains achieved with Phases I and II.

Phase IV

The functional restoration and maintenance phase of rehabilitation was often neglected in the past. It is the basis for today's sport-specific training in sports medicine and involves the practice and analysis of functional tasks that are similar to those used during sport activities (i.e., throwing or hitting a tennis ball), as well as correcting any biomechanical deficits that may occur during such activities. The main purpose of this phase is to reduce the likelihood of reinjury while attaining the previous level of function. Phase IV is initiated when the involved joint or muscle has attained from 80 to 90 percent of normal strength and painless range of motion as compared to the contralateral side.

Chapter 33

Heat Illness

Understanding warm and/or hot weather definitions is very important for an athlete or just an exerciser for fitness so that they may better comprehend heat illness, preventative measures, and treatment options if necessary. Of the many relevant heat-related definitions, the heat index is one of the most important.

Steadman or Heat Index: The combination of air temperature and humidity that gives a description of how the temperature feels. This is not the actual air temperature. When the heat index is at or over 90 degrees Fahrenheit, extreme caution should be considered before exercising outdoors.

Heat Illness: What Is It And How Do You Manage It?

Heat illness or exertional heat illness progresses along a continuum from the mild (heat rash and/or heat cramps and/or heat syncope) through the moderate (heat exhaustion) to the life-threatening (heatstroke). Anyone is susceptible to a heat-related exertional illness. It is very important that the athlete or exerciser understand that the presentation of signs and symptoms associated with heat exertional illness does not necessarily follow this continuum. A dehydrated, nonacclimated or deconditioned individual may right away present with signs and symptoms consistent with heat stroke and not the milder symptoms first.

Heat Cramps are associated with excessive sweating during exercise and are usually caused by dehydration, electrolyte (primarily salt) loss, and inadequate blood flow to the peripheral muscles. They usually occur in the quadriceps, hamstrings, and calves.

About This Chapter: This chapter includes text excerpted from "Exercising In Hot Weather," U.S. Public Health Service Commissioned Corps (PHSCC), U.S. Department of Health and Human Services (HHS), August 5, 2007. Reviewed July 2017.

Treatment for heat cramps is rehydration with an electrolyte (salt) solution and muscle stretch.

Heat Syncope results from physical exertion in a hot environment. In an effort to increase heat loss, the skin blood vessels dilate to such an extent that blood flow to the brain is reduced causing symptoms of headache, dizziness, faintness, increased heart rate, nausea, vomiting, restlessness, and possibly even a brief loss of consciousness.

Treatment for heat syncope is to sit or lie down in a cool environment with elevation of the feet. Hydration is very important so there is not a possible progression to heat exhaustion or heat stroke.

Heat Exhaustion is a shock-like condition that occurs when excessive sweating causes dehydration and electrolyte loss. A person with heat exhaustion may have headache, nausea, dizziness, chills, fatigue, and extreme thirst. Signs of heat exhaustion are pale and clammy skin, rapid and weak pulse, loss of coordination, decreased performance, dilated pupils, and profuse sweating.

Treatment for heat exhaustion is to immediately stop the activity and properly hydrate with chilled water and/or an electrolyte replacement sport beverage. The exerciser should be cleared by his/her physician before resuming sport or other strenuous outdoor activities.

Hydration

Ideally you want to stay hydrated while training. You must take in roughly the same amount of fluid you lose in sweat to maintain hydration. It is a good idea to drink fluids throughout the day, including before, during and after sports and exercise.

Water is probably the best beverage for most people. For intense heat or longer training sessions, drinks with sodium and electrolytes can help restore fluids.

For athletes training or competing over many days, weighing yourself daily can help you determine if you are adequately replacing lost fluids.

(Source: "Tips For Practicing And Competing In Hot And Humid Conditions For Athletes," Office of Disease Prevention and Health Promotion (ODPHP), U.S. Department of Health and Human Services (HHS).)

Exertional Heat Stroke (Hyperthermia) is a life-threatening condition in which the body's thermal regulatory mechanism is overwhelmed. There are two types heat stroke—fluid depleted (slow onset) and fluid intact (fast onset). Fluid depleted means that the individual is not hydrating at a rate sufficient to function in a heat challenge situation. Fluid intact means that the extreme heat overwhelms the individual even though the fluid level is sufficient. Key signs of heat stroke are hot skin (not necessarily dry skin), peripheral vasoconstriction (pale or ashen colored skin), high pulse rate, high respiratory rate, decreased urine output, and a core temperature (taken rectally) over 104 or 105 degrees Fahrenheit, and pupils may be dilated and unresponsive to light.

Treatment for heat stroke is to move the person to a cool shaded area and reduce the body temperature immediately. If immediate medical attention is not available, immerse the person in a cool bath while covering the extremities with cool wet cloths and massaging the extremities to propel the cooled blood back into the core.

Cooling Measures

Many options to cool your body before and during activity exist. Precooling your body with ice towels before you train or compete is one option. Fans, ice vests, and even cold baths can help athletes in extreme conditions.

(Source: "Tips For Practicing And Competing In Hot And Humid Conditions For Athletes," Office of Disease Prevention and Health Promotion (ODPHP), U.S. Department of Health and Human Services (HHS).)

Exercise-Induced Hyponatremia (Water Intoxication) is most commonly associated with prolonged exertion during sustained, high-intensity endurance activities such as marathons or triathlons. In most cases, it is attributable to excess free water intake, which fails to replenish the sometimes massive sodium losses that result from sweating. Symptoms of hyponatremia can vary from light-headedness, malaise, nausea, to altered mental status. Risk factors include hot weather, female athletes/exercisers, poor performance, and possibly the use of nonsteroidal anti-inflammatory medications.

As a treatment for hyponatremia, new guidelines advise runners to drink only as much fluid as they lose due to sweating during a race. The International Marathon Medical Directors Association (IMMDA) recommends that, during extended exercise, athletes drink no more than 31 ounces (or about 800 milliliters) of water per hour. Individuals involved in strenuous exercise in warm or hot weather should consider the sodium (salt) concentration of the beverage being consumed.

How Can You Prevent Exertional Heat-Related Illnesses?

Some recommendations on how to prevent exertional heat-related illness include:

- When exercising in high heat and humidity, rest 10 minutes for every hour and change wet clothing frequently.

191

- Avoid the midday sun by exercising before 10 a.m. or after 6 p.m., if possible.

- Use a sunscreen with a rating of SPF (sun protection factor)-15 or lower dependent upon skin type. Ratings above SPF-15 can interfere with the skin's thermal regulation.

- Wear light-weight and breathable clothing.

- Weigh yourself pre- and post-exercise. If there is a less than a 2 percent weight loss after exercise, you are considered mildly dehydrated. With a 2 percent and greater weight loss, you are considered dehydrated.

- During hot weather training, dehydration occurs more frequently and has more severe consequences. Drink early and at regular intervals according to the American College of Sports Medicine (ACSM). The perception of thirst is a poor index of the magnitude of fluid deficit. Monitoring your weight loss and ingesting chilled volumes of fluid during exercise at a rate equal to that lost from sweating is a better method to preventing dehydration.

- Rapid fluid replacement is not recommended for rehydration. Rapid replacement of fluid stimulates increased urine production, which reduces the body water retention.

- Individuals involved in a short bout of exercise are generally fine with water fluid replacement of an extra 8–16 ounces. A sports drink (with salt and potassium) is suggested for exercise lasting longer than an hour, such as a marathon, and at a rate of about 16 to 24 ounces an hour depending upon the amount you sweat and the heat index.

- Replace fluids after long bouts of exercise (greater than an hour) at a rate of 16 ounces of fluid per pound of body weight lost during exercise.

- Avoid caffeinated, protein, and alcoholic drinks, e.g., colored soda, coffee, tea.

- Acclimate to exercising outdoors, altitude, and physical condition. General rule of thumb is 10–14 days for adults and 14–21 days for children (prepubescent) and older adults (> 60 years). Children and older adults are less heat tolerant and have a less effective thermoregulatory system.

- Educate and prepare yourself for outdoor activities. Many websites offer heat index calculations for your local weather conditions. Two websites that will calculate the heat index for you are www.erh.noaa.gov/box/calculate2.html and www.compuweather.com/shared/weather_calculator.htm.

Weather does not have to sideline your outdoor exercise regimen. The above suggestions can help you plan and find ways to modify your routine to exercise safely in warm, hot, and humid weather.

Chapter 34

Sprains And Strains

What Is The Difference Between A Sprain And A Strain?

A sprain is a stretch and/or tear of a ligament (a band of fibrous tissue that connects two or more bones at a joint). One or more ligaments can be injured at the same time. The severity of the injury will depend on the extent of injury (whether a tear is partial or complete) and the number of ligaments involved.

A strain is an injury to either a muscle or a tendon (fibrous cords of tissue that connect muscle to bone). Depending on the severity of the injury, a strain may be a simple overstretch of the muscle or tendon, or it can result from a partial or complete tear.

What Causes A Sprain?

A sprain can result from a fall, a sudden twist, or a blow to the body that forces a joint out of its normal position and stretches or tears the ligament supporting that joint. Typically, sprains occur when people fall and land on an outstretched arm, slide into a baseball base, land on the side of their foot, or twist a knee with the foot planted firmly on the ground.

Where Do Sprains Usually Occur?

Although sprains can occur in both the upper and lower parts of the body, the most common site is the ankle. It is estimated that more than 628,000 ankle sprains occur in the United States each year.

About This Chapter: This chapter includes text excerpted from "Questions And Answers About Sprains And Strains," National Institute of Arthritis and Musculoskeletal and Skin Diseases (NIAMS), January 2015.

The ankle joint is supported by several lateral (outside) ligaments and medial (inside) ligaments (see figure 34.1). Most ankle sprains happen when the foot turns inward as a person runs, turns, falls, or lands on the ankle after a jump. This type of sprain is called an inversion injury. The knee is another common site for a sprain. A blow to the knee or a fall is often the cause; sudden twisting can also result in a sprain (see figure 34.2).

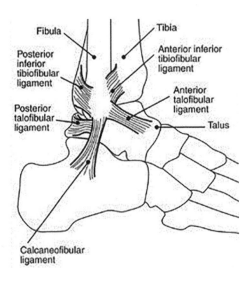

Figure 34.1. Lateral View Of The Ankle

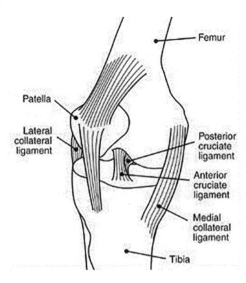

Figure 34.2. Lateral View Of The Knee

Sprains frequently occur at the wrist, typically when people fall and land on an outstretched hand. A sprain to the thumb is common in skiing and other sports. This injury often occurs when a ligament near the base of the thumb (the ulnar collateral ligament of the metacarpophalangeal joint) is torn (see figure 34.3).

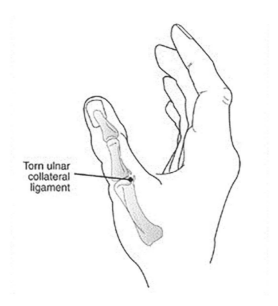

Torn ulnar collateral ligament

Figure 34.3. Lateral View Of The Thumb

What Are The Signs And Symptoms Of A Sprain?

The usual signs and symptoms include pain, swelling, bruising, instability, and loss of the ability to move and use the joint (called functional ability). However, these signs and symptoms can vary in intensity, depending on the severity of the sprain. Sometimes people feel a pop or tear when the injury happens.

Doctors closely observe an injured site and ask questions to obtain information to diagnose the severity of a sprain. In general, a grade I or mild sprain is caused by overstretching or slight tearing of the ligaments with no joint instability. A person with a mild sprain usually experiences minimal pain, swelling, and little or no loss of functional ability. Bruising is absent or slight, and the person is usually able to put weight on the affected joint.

A grade II or moderate sprain is caused by further, but still incomplete, tearing of the ligament and is characterized by bruising, moderate pain, and swelling. A person with a moderate sprain usually has more difficulty putting weight on the affected joint and experiences some loss of function. An X-ray may be needed to help the healthcare provider determine if a fracture is causing the pain and swelling. Magnetic resonance imaging is occasionally used to help differentiate between a significant partial injury and a complete tear in a ligament, or can be recommended to rule out other injuries.

People who sustain a grade III or severe sprain completely tear or rupture a ligament. Pain, swelling, and bruising are usually severe, and the patient is unable to put weight on the joint. An X-ray is usually taken to rule out a broken bone. When diagnosing any sprain, the healthcare provider will ask the patient to explain how the injury happened. He or she will examine the affected area and check its stability and its ability to move and bear weight.

When To See A Healthcare Provider For A Sprain

- You have severe pain and cannot put any weight on the injured joint.
- The injured area looks crooked or has lumps and bumps (other than swelling) that you do not see on the uninjured joint.
- You cannot move the injured joint.
- You cannot walk more than four steps without significant pain.
- Your limb buckles or gives way when you try to use the joint.
- You have numbness in any part of the injured area.
- You see redness or red streaks spreading out from the injury.
- You injure an area that has been injured several times before.
- You have pain, swelling, or redness over a bony part of your foot.
- You are in doubt about the seriousness of the injury or how to care for it.

What Causes A Strain?

A strain is caused by twisting or pulling a muscle or tendon. Strains can be acute or chronic. An acute strain is associated with a recent trauma or injury; it also can occur after improperly lifting heavy objects or overstressing the muscles. Chronic strains are usually the result of overuse: prolonged, repetitive movement of the muscles and tendons.

Where Do Strains Usually Occur?

Two common sites for a strain are the back and the hamstring muscle (located in the back of the thigh). Contact sports such as soccer, football, hockey, boxing, and wrestling put people at risk for strains. Gymnastics, tennis, rowing, golf, and other sports that require extensive gripping can increase the risk of hand and forearm strains. Elbow strains sometimes occur in people who participate in racquet sports, throwing, and contact sports.

What Are The Signs And Symptoms Of A Strain?

Typically, people with a strain experience pain, limited motion, muscle spasms, and possibly muscle weakness. They also can have localized swelling, cramping, or inflammation and, with a minor or moderate strain, usually some loss of muscle function. Patients typically have pain in the injured area and general weakness of the muscle when they attempt to move it. Severe strains that partially or completely tear the muscle or tendon are often very painful and disabling.

How Are Sprains And Strains Treated?
Reduce Swelling And Pain

Treatments for sprains and strains are similar and can be thought of as having two stages. The goal during the first stage is to reduce swelling and pain. At this stage, healthcare providers

---

RICE Therapy
Rest

Reduce regular exercise or activities of daily living as needed. Your healthcare provider may advise you to put no weight on an injured area for 48 hours. If you cannot put weight on an ankle or knee, crutches may help. If you use a cane or one crutch for an ankle injury, use it on the uninjured side to help you lean away and relieve weight on the injured ankle.

Ice

Apply an ice pack to the injured area for 20 minutes at a time, four to eight times a day. A cold pack, ice bag, or plastic bag filled with crushed ice and wrapped in a towel can be used. To avoid cold injury and frostbite, do not apply the ice for more than 20 minutes.

Compression

Compression of an injured ankle, knee, or wrist may help reduce swelling. Examples of compression bandages are elastic wraps, special boots, air casts, and splints. Ask your healthcare provider for advice on which one to use and how tight to apply the bandage safely.

Elevation

If possible, keep the injured ankle, knee, elbow, or wrist elevated on a pillow, above the level of the heart, to help decrease swelling.

---

usually advise patients to follow a formula of rest, ice, compression, and elevation (RICE) for the first 24 to 48 hours after the injury. The healthcare provider also may recommend an over-the-counter or prescription medication to help decrease pain and inflammation.

For people with a moderate or severe sprain, particularly of the ankle, a hard cast may be applied. This often occurs after the initial swelling has subsided. Severe sprains and strains may require surgery to repair the torn ligaments, muscle, or tendons. Surgery is usually performed by an orthopaedic surgeon.

It is important that moderate and severe sprains and strains be evaluated by a healthcare provider to allow prompt, appropriate treatment to begin. This box lists some signs that should alert people to consult their healthcare provider. However, a person who has any concerns about the seriousness of a sprain or strain should always contact a healthcare provider for advice.

Begin Rehabilitation

The second stage of treating a sprain or strain is rehabilitation, with the overall goal of improving the condition of the injured area and restoring its function. The healthcare provider will prescribe an exercise program designed to prevent stiffness, improve range of motion, and restore the joint's normal flexibility and strength. Some patients may need physical therapy during this stage. When the acute pain and swelling have diminished, the healthcare provider will instruct the patient to do a series of exercises several times a day. These are very important because they help reduce swelling, prevent stiffness, and restore normal, pain-free range of motion. The healthcare provider can recommend many different types of exercises, depending on the injury. A patient with an injured knee or foot will work on weight-bearing and balancing exercises. The duration of the program depends on the extent of the injury, but the regimen commonly lasts for several weeks.

Another goal of rehabilitation is to increase strength and regain flexibility. Depending on the patient's rate of recovery, this process begins about the second week after the injury. The healthcare provider will instruct the patient to do a series of exercises designed to meet these goals. During this phase of rehabilitation, patients progress to more demanding exercises as pain decreases and function improves.

The final goal is the return to full daily activities, including sports when appropriate. Patients must work closely with their healthcare provider or physical therapist to determine their readiness to return to full activity. Sometimes people are tempted to resume full activity or play sports despite pain or muscle soreness. Returning to full activity before regaining normal range of motion, flexibility, and strength increases the chance of reinjury and may lead to a chronic problem.

The amount of rehabilitation and the time needed for full recovery after a sprain or strain depend on the severity of the injury and individual rates of healing. For example, a mild ankle sprain may require 3 to 6 weeks of rehabilitation; a moderate sprain could require 2 to 3 months. With a severe sprain, it can take 8 to 12 months to return to full activities. Extra care should be taken to avoid reinjury.

Can Sprains And Strains Be Prevented?

People can do many things to help lower their risk of sprains and strains:

- Avoid exercising or playing sports when tired or in pain.

- Maintain a healthy, well-balanced diet to keep muscles strong.

- Maintain a healthy weight.

- Practice safety measures to help prevent falls. For example, keep stairways, walkways, yards, and driveways free of clutter; anchor scatter rugs; and salt or sand icy sidewalks and driveways in the winter.

- Wear shoes that fit properly.

- Replace athletic shoes as soon as the tread wears out or the heel wears down on one side.

- Do stretching exercises daily.

- Be in proper physical condition to play a sport.

- Warm up and stretch before participating in any sport or exercise.

- Wear protective equipment when playing.

- Run on even surfaces.

Chapter 35

Broken Bones

Sports-related injuries such as bruises, scrapes, and broken bones accounted for 22 percent of hospital emergency department visits for children ages 5 to 17 in 2006, according to the latest News and Numbers from the Agency for Healthcare Research and Quality (AHRQ).

The Federal agency's analysis also shows that in 2006:

- Boys had 3 times more visits to treat sports injuries than did girls (147 visits per 10,000 children versus 50 visits per 10,000 children).

- Teens were 5 times more likely than children to be treated for sports injuries in emergency departments (154 visits per 10,000 15 to 17 year-olds versus 30 visits per 10,000 5 to 9 year-olds).

- Some 81 percent of all visits were for bruises, sprains and strains, arm fractures, or cuts and scrapes to the head, neck, or chest.

- Only 1.3 percent of visits resulted in hospital admissions, mostly for leg and arm fractures. In nearly 99 percent of visits, the children were treated and released.

Why Are Broken Bones Dangerous?

Broken bones can cause serious health problems:

- The most common bones that break are the hip, wrist, and spine (backbone).

About This Chapter: Text in this chapter begins with excerpts from "Sports Injuries Caused 1 In 5 Emergency Department Visits For Kids," Agency for Healthcare Research and Quality (AHRQ), U.S. Department of Health and Human Services (HHS), July 1, 2009. Reviewed July 2017; Text beginning with the heading "Why Are Broken Bones Dangerous?" is excerpted from "Reducing The Risk Of Bone Fracture," Effective Health Care (EHC) Program, Agency for Healthcare Research and Quality (AHRQ), May 2012. Reviewed July 2017; Text beginning with the heading "First Aid" is © 2017 Omnigraphics. Reviewed July 2017.

- Broken bones can cause ongoing pain and make it hard to do daily activities.

- The bones in your spine can crunch together and cause pain. This could cause you to lose an inch or more of height.

- While recovering from a broken bone—especially the hip—you may need constant care and may have to stay in a nursing home.

- If you break your hip, you will probably need surgery to fix it. Surgery increases your risk for other health problems.

- Once you break a bone, you may be more likely to break other bones, which could lead to more health problems.

What Treatments Can Help Lower The Risk Of Breaking A Bone?

For people with low bone density, there are treatments that can help strengthen bones and lower the risk of breaking a bone. Your doctor may suggest one or more of the following treatments:

- Medicines

- Nutritional Supplements

- Exercise

What Medicines Are Available?

Medicines that help reduce the risk of breaking a bone either help slow the breakdown of old bone or help build new bone more quickly.

- Most research has been done to see how well these medicines work for women with osteoporosis who have already gone through menopause. Not as many studies have been done to see if these medicines work for men or for women who have not gone through menopause.

- Some of these medicines may also be taken by people with osteopenia.

- There is not enough research to exactly know how much the medicines will lower the risk of breaking a bone.

- Even if your bone density does not change while you are taking medicine, that does not mean the medicine is not working to protect you from breaking a bone.

Can Nutritional Supplements Help Keep My Bones Healthy?

Your doctor may recommend you take calcium and vitamin D alone or with your prescription medicines to help strengthen your bones and lower your risk of developing osteoporosis. Researchers are not sure if taking calcium or vitamin D without other treatment reduces the risk of breaking a bone for people with osteoporosis.

Your body needs calcium to build bones, and vitamin D helps your body use calcium. The amount of calcium and vitamin D you need each day depends on your age.

It is important to make sure your diet is high in calcium and vitamin D. You can get calcium and vitamin D from many foods. Your doctor may recommend you buy pills (prescription or over-the-counter) that contain calcium and vitamin D. Talk with your doctor about how much calcium and vitamin D is right for you.

Sources of calcium include:

- Dairy foods like milk, cheese, and yogurt.

- Dark green leafy vegetables like broccoli and kale.

- Bread, pasta, cereal, and rice contain low amounts of calcium.

- Foods that are "fortified" with calcium (contain added calcium), like many fruit juices, tofu, and cereals.

Sources of vitamin D include:

- Fatty fish like salmon, tuna, and mackerel.

- Green leafy vegetables.

- Beef liver and egg yolks provide a small amount of vitamin D.

- Foods fortified with vitamin D, like milk, cereal, some fruit juices, and yogurt.

- Sunlight.

Can Exercise Help?

Your doctor may also recommend exercises to help strengthen your bones, improve your balance, and reduce your chance of falling.

- "Weight-bearing" exercises use extra weight and gravity to make bones stronger.

- Weight-bearing exercises include walking, lifting weights, and climbing stairs.

- Some exercises may be too hard on your bones and can increase your risk of breaking a bone. For example, activities like golf require you to twist your body in ways that might be dangerous.

- Talk with your doctor about what exercises are best for you.

What Should I Think About When Deciding?

Only you and your doctor can decide whether any medicine's ability to help your condition is worth the risk of a serious side effect. Each person responds differently to different medicines. Your doctor may try several medicines before finding the right one.

There are several things to consider when deciding which treatment might be best for you:

- If you have osteopenia (mild low bone density), whether you need to start medicines now or can wait and see if your condition gets worse.

- What your bone density test says is your risk for breaking a bone.

- The benefits and side effects of each treatment.

- Ways your doctor can help you notice any side effects so they can be treated or the medicine can be changed.

- Which medicine best fits your daily life and routine.

- The out-of-pocket costs of each treatment option, and whether medicines come in generic form.

First Aid

Providing first aid when a break first occurs plays a key role in the treatment of broken bones. It can prevent any further damage and thereby may decrease recovery time. Those providing first aid for a broken bone should:

- **Stop any bleeding:** If the injured athlete is bleeding, apply pressure to the wound using a sterile bandage or a clean cloth.

- **Restrict movement:** If the athlete has suffered a fracture, restrict movement of the limb or other body part using a sling or splint to avoid further damage.

- **Ice pack:** Apply an ice pack to the injured area to reduce swelling and pain.

Treatment

Broken bones are generally treated by putting the broken pieces back in to position and allowing them to heal by restricting further movement in place. Some ways in which broken bones are treated include:

- **Casting And Bracing**

  Casting is the most commonly used form of treatment for fractures. Broken bones are placed in proper position and a cast of plaster or fiberglass is applied to help it heal.

  In some cases, doctors can use a brace or a functional cast that allows the athlete some movement of the limb or related joints. However, not all fractures can be treated in this manner and most will need complete immobilization.

- **External And Internal Fixation**

  Certain fractures will need additional support to remain in alignment while the bones to heal. If the skin over a fracture is badly damaged or the patient is still growing, doctors may use an external fixation device. Metal pins or screws are placed into fractured bones and then connected to a metal bar outside of the skin that keeps the fractured bones in proper position. Once the skin and muscle around the bone is healed, physicians may then perform an operation referred to as open reduction and internal fixation.

In open reduction and internal fixation, the surgeon will access the bone fragments and realign them properly. The surgeon will then attach screws and metal plates to the bone surface, or insert a metal rod into the center of the fractured bone, to hold the pieces in place.

Recovery

A fracture may take weeks if not months to heal completely and care must be taken to ensure completer healing. Follow your doctor's instructions carefully, particularly in regard to moving or placing weight on the fractured bone. Doctor will also subsequently prescribe physical therapy to strengthen weakened muscles and joints around the fracture and to restore range of motion.

References

1. "First Aid For Broken Bones And Fractures," Healthline Media, October 17, 2016.

2. "Fractures (Broken Bones)," American Academy of Orthopaedic Surgeons (AAOS), October 2012.

Chapter 36

Growth Plate Injuries

What Is The Growth Plate?

The growth plate, also known as the epiphyseal plate or physis, is the area of growing tissue near the ends of the long bones in children and adolescents. Each long bone has at least two growth plates: one at each end. The growth plate determines the future length and shape of the mature bone. When growth is complete—sometime during adolescence—the growth plates close and are replaced by solid bone.

Because the growth plates are the weakest areas of the growing skeleton—even weaker than the nearby ligaments and tendons that connect bones to other bones and muscles—they are vulnerable to injury. Injuries to the growth plate are called fractures.

Who Gets Growth Plate Injuries?

Growth plate injuries can occur in growing children and adolescents. In a child, a serious injury to a joint is more likely to damage a growth plate than the ligaments that stabilize the joint. Trauma that would cause a sprain in an adult might cause a growth plate fracture in a child.

Growth plate fractures occur twice as often in boys as in girls, because girls' bodies mature at an earlier age than boys. As a result, their bones finish growing sooner, and their growth plates are replaced by stronger, solid bone.

About This Chapter: This chapter includes text excerpted from "Growth Plate Injuries—Questions And Answers About Growth Plate Injuries," National Institute of Arthritis and Musculoskeletal and Skin Diseases (NIAMS), May 2014.

Growth plate injuries often occur in competitive sports such as football, basketball, or gymnastics, or as a result of recreational activities such as biking, sledding, skiing, or skateboarding.

Fractures can result from a single traumatic event, such as a fall or automobile accident, or from chronic stress and overuse. Most growth plate fractures occur in the long bones of the fingers (phalanges) and the outer bone of the forearm (radius). They are also common in the lower bones of the leg (the tibia and fibula).

What Causes Growth Plate Injuries?

Growth plate injuries can be caused by an event such as a fall or blow to the limb, or they can result from overuse. For example, a gymnast who practices for hours on the uneven bars, a long-distance runner, and a baseball pitcher perfecting his curveball can all have growth plate injuries.

Although many growth plate injuries are caused by accidents that occur during play or athletic activity, growth plates are also susceptible to other disorders, such as bone infection, that can alter their normal growth and development. Other possible causes of growth plate injuries include the following:

- **Child abuse.** Fractures are common among physically abused children, and growth plate injuries are prevalent because the growth plate is the weakest part of the bone.

- **Injury from extreme cold (for example, frostbite).** Exposure to extreme cold can damage the growth plate in children and result in short, stubby fingers or premature degenerative arthritis (breakdown of the joint cartilage).

- **Radiation and medications.** Research has suggested that chemotherapy given for childhood cancers may negatively affect bone growth. Prolonged use of steroids for inflammatory conditions such as juvenile idiopathic arthritis can also harm bone growth.

- **Neurological disorders.** Children with certain neurological disorders that result in sensory deficit or muscular imbalance are prone to growth plate fractures, especially at the ankle and knee. Children who are born with insensitivity to pain can have similar types of injuries.

- **Genetics.** The growth plates are where many inherited disorders that affect the musculoskeletal system appear. Scientists are beginning to understand the genes and gene mutations involved in skeletal formation, growth, and development. This new information is raising hopes for improving treatment for children who are born with poorly formed or improperly functioning growth plates.

- **Metabolic disease.** Disease states such as kidney failure and hormone disorders can affect the growth plates and their function. The bone growth of children with long-term conditions of this kind may be negatively affected.

How Are Growth Plate Fractures Diagnosed?

A child who has persistent pain, or pain that affects athletic performance or the ability to move and put pressure on a limb, should never be allowed or expected to "work through the pain." Whether an injury is acute or due to overuse, it should be evaluated by a doctor, because some injuries, if left untreated, can cause permanent damage and interfere with proper growth of the involved limb.

The doctor will begin the diagnostic process by asking about the injury and how it occurred and by examining the child. The doctor will then use X-rays to determine if there is a fracture, and if so, the type of fracture. Often the doctor will X-ray not only the injured limb but the opposite limb as well. Because growth plates have not yet hardened into solid bone, neither the structures themselves nor injuries to them show up on X-rays. Instead, growth plates appear as gaps between the shaft of a long bone, called the metaphysis, and the end of the bone, called the epiphysis. By comparing X-rays of the injured limb to those of the noninjured limb, doctors can look for differences that indicate an injury.

Very often the X-ray is negative, because the growth plate line is already there, and the fracture is undisplaced (the two ends of the broken bone are not separated). The doctor can still diagnose a growth plate fracture on clinical grounds because of tenderness of the plate. Children do get ligament strains if their growth plates are open, and they often have undisplaced growth plate fractures.

Other tests doctors may use to diagnose a growth plate injury include magnetic resonance imaging (MRI), computed tomography (CT), and ultrasound.

Because these tests enable doctors to see the growth plate and areas of other soft tissue, they can be useful not only in detecting the presence of an injury, but also in determining the type and extent of the injury.

What Are The Different Types Of Growth Plate Injuries?

Since the 1960s, the Salter-Harris classification, which divides most growth plate fractures into five categories based on the type of damage, has been the standard. The categories are as follows:

Type I: Fracture Through The Growth Plate

The epiphysis is completely separated from the end of the bone or the metaphysis, through the deep layer of the growth plate. The growth plate remains attached to the epiphysis. The doctor has to put the fracture back into place if it is significantly displaced. Type I injuries generally require a cast to protect the plate as it heals. Unless there is damage to the blood supply to the growth plate, the likelihood that the bone will grow normally is excellent.

Type II: Fracture Through The Growth Plate And Metaphysis

This is the most common type of growth plate fracture. It runs through the growth plate and the metaphysis, but the epiphysis is not involved in the injury. Like type I fractures, type II fractures may need to be put back into place and immobilized. However, the growth plate fracture heals a great deal, especially in younger children. If it is not too displaced, the doctor may not need to put it back into position. In this case, it will strengthen with time.

Type III: Fracture Through Growth Plate And Epiphysis

This fracture occurs only rarely, usually at the lower end of the tibia, one of the long bones of the lower leg. It happens when a fracture runs completely through the epiphysis and separates part of the epiphysis and growth plate from the metaphysis. Surgery is sometimes necessary to restore the joint surface to normal. The outlook or prognosis for growth is good if the blood supply to the separated portion of the epiphysis is still intact and if the joint surface heals in a normal position.

Type IV: Fracture Through Growth Plate, Metaphysis, And Epiphysis

This fracture runs through the epiphysis, across the growth plate, and into the metaphysis. Surgery is frequently needed to restore the joint surface to normal and to perfectly align the growth plate. Unless perfect alignment is achieved and maintained during healing, prognosis for growth is poor, and angulation (bending) of the bone may occur. This injury occurs most commonly at the end of the humerus (the upper arm bone) near the elbow.

Type V: Compression Fracture Through Growth Plate

This uncommon injury occurs when the end of the bone is crushed and the growth plate is compressed. It is most likely to occur at the knee or ankle. Prognosis is poor, since premature stunting of growth is almost inevitable.

A newer classification, called the Peterson classification, adds a type VI fracture, in which a portion of the epiphysis, growth plate, and metaphysis is missing. This usually occurs with open wounds or compound fractures, and often involves lawnmowers, farm machinery, snow-mobiles, or gunshot wounds. All type VI fractures require surgery, and most will require later reconstructive or corrective surgery. Bone growth is almost always stunted.

What Kind Of Doctor Treats Growth Plate Injuries?

For all but the simplest injuries, the child's doctor will probably refer him or her to an orthopaedic surgeon (a doctor who specializes in bone and joint problems in children and adults) for treatment. Some problems may require the services of a pediatric orthopaedic surgeon, who specializes in injuries and musculoskeletal disorders in children.

How Are Growth Plate Injuries Treated?

Treatment for growth plate injuries depends on the type of injury. In all cases, treatment should be started as soon as possible after injury and will generally involve a mix of the following:

Immobilization

The affected limb is often put in a cast or splint, and the child is told to limit any activity that puts pressure on the injured area.

Manipulation Or Surgery

If the fracture is displaced (meaning the ends of the injured bones no longer meet as they should), the doctor will have to put the bones or joints back in their correct positions, either by using his or her hands (called manipulation) or by performing surgery. Sometimes the doctor needs to fix the break and hold the growth plate in place with screws or wire. After the procedure, the bone will be set in place (immobilized) so it can heal without moving. This is usually done with a cast that encloses the injured growth plate and the joints on both sides of it. The cast is left in place until the injury heals, which can take anywhere from a few weeks to 2 or more months for serious injuries. The need for manipulation or surgery depends on the location and extent of the injury, its effect on nearby nerves and blood vessels, and the child's age.

Strengthening And Range-Of-Motion Exercises

These are exercises designed to strengthen the muscles that support the injured area of the bone and to improve or maintain the joint's ability to move in the way that it should.

Your child's doctor may recommend these after the fracture has healed. A physical therapist can work with the child and his or her doctor to design an appropriate exercise plan. Long-term followup is usually necessary to monitor the child's recuperation and growth.

Will The Affected Limb Of A Child With A Growth Plate Injury Still Grow?

Most growth plate fractures heal without any lasting effect. Whether an arrest of growth occurs depends on the treatment provided, and the following factors, in descending order of importance:

- **Severity of the injury.** If the injury causes the blood supply to the epiphysis to be cut off, growth can be stunted. If the growth plate is shifted, shattered, or crushed, the growth plate may close prematurely, forming a bony bridge or "bar." The risk of growth arrest is higher in this setting. An open injury in which the skin is broken carries the risk of infection, which could destroy the growth plate.

- **Age of the child.** In a younger child, the bones have a great deal of growing to do; therefore, growth arrest can be more serious, and closer surveillance is needed. It is also true, however, that younger bones have a greater ability to heal.

- **Which growth plate is injured.** Some growth plates, such as those in the region of the knee, are more involved in extensive bone growth than others.

- **Type of fracture.** Of the six fracture types described earlier, types IV, V, and VI are the most serious.

The most frequent complication of a growth plate fracture is premature arrest of bone growth. The affected bone grows less than it would have without the injury, and the resulting limb could be shorter than the opposite, uninjured limb. If only part of the growth plate is injured, growth may be lopsided and the limb may become crooked.

Growth plate injuries at the knee have the greatest risk of complications. Nerve and blood vessel damage occurs most frequently there. Injuries to the knee have a much higher incidence of premature growth arrest and crooked growth.

Chapter 37

Concussions

A concussion is a type of traumatic brain injury—or TBI—caused by a bump, blow, or jolt to the head or by a hit to the body that causes the head and brain to move rapidly back and forth. This sudden movement can cause the brain to bounce around or twist in the skull, creating chemical changes in the brain and sometimes stretching and damaging brain cells.

Concussions Are Serious

Medical providers may describe a concussion as a "mild" brain injury because concussions are usually not life-threatening. Even so, the effects of a concussion can be serious.

Concussion Signs And Symptoms

Children and teens who show or report one or more of the signs and symptoms listed below, or simply say they just "don't feel right" after a bump, blow, or jolt to the head or body, may have a concussion or more serious brain injury.

Concussion Signs Observed

- Can't recall events prior to or after a hit or fall.

- Appears dazed or stunned.

- Forgets an instruction, is confused about an assignment or position, or is unsure of the game, score, or opponent.

About This Chapter: This chapter includes text excerpted from "Brain Injury Basics—What Is A Concussion?" Centers for Disease Control and Prevention (CDC), January 31, 2017.

- Moves clumsily.

- Answers questions slowly.

- Loses consciousness (even briefly).

- Shows mood, behavior, or personality changes.

Concussion Symptoms Reported

- Headache or "pressure" in head.

- Nausea or vomiting.

- Balance problems or dizziness, or double or blurry vision.

- Bothered by light or noise.

- Feeling sluggish, hazy, foggy, or groggy.

- Confusion, or concentration or memory problems.

- Just not "feeling right," or "feeling down."

Signs and symptoms generally show up soon after the injury. However, children may not know how serious the injury is at first and some symptoms may not show up for hours or days. For example, in the first few minutes a child or a teen might be little confused or a bit dazed, but an hour later the child might not be able to remember how he or she got hurt.

Parents should continue to check for signs of concussion right after the injury and a few days after the injury. If the child or teen's concussion signs or symptoms get worse, parents should take him or her to the emergency department right away.

Concussion Danger Signs

In rare cases, a dangerous collection of blood (hematoma) may form on the brain after a bump, blow, or jolt to the head or body that may squeeze the brain against the skull. Call 9-1-1 right away, or take the child or teen to the emergency department if he or she has one or more of the following danger signs after a bump, blow, or jolt to the head or body:

Dangerous Signs And Symptoms Of A Concussion

- One pupil larger than the other.

- Drowsiness or inability to wake up.

- A headache that gets worse and does not go away.

- Slurred speech, weakness, numbness, or decreased coordination.

- Repeated vomiting or nausea, convulsions or seizures (shaking or twitching).

- Unusual behavior, increased confusion, restlessness, or agitation.

- Loss of consciousness (passed out/knocked out). Even a brief loss of consciousness should be taken seriously.

Severe Brain Injury

Long-Term Effects

A person with a severe brain injury will need to be hospitalized and may have long-term problems affecting things such as:

- Thinking

- Memory

- Learning

- Coordination and balance

- Speech, hearing or vision

- Emotions

A severe brain injury can affect all aspects of people's lives, including relationships with family and friends, as well as their ability to work or be employed, do household chores, drive, and/or do other normal daily activities.

Recovery From Concussion

Rest is very important after a concussion because it helps the brain heal. The child or teen may need to limit activities while he or she is recovering from a concussion. Physical activities or activities that involve a lot of concentration, such as studying, working on the computer, or playing video games may cause concussion symptoms (such as headache or tiredness) to come back or get worse. After a concussion, physical and cognitive activities—such as concentration and learning—should be carefully watched by a medical provider. As the days go by, the child or teen can expect to slowly feel better.

Postconcussive Syndrome

While most children and teens with a concussion feel better within a couple of weeks, some will have symptoms for months or longer. Talk with the healthcare provider if their concussion symptoms do not go away or if they get worse after they return to their regular activities.

> One common but misleading claim: Using a particular dietary supplement promotes faster healing after a concussion or other TBI.
>
> Even if a particular supplement contains no harmful ingredients, that claim alone can be dangerous, says Gary Coody, U.S. Food and Drug Administration's (FDA) National Health Fraud Coordinator.
>
> *(Source: "Can A Dietary Supplement Treat A Concussion? No!" U.S. Food and Drug Administration (FDA).)*

Returning To Sports And Activities

After a concussion, an athlete should only return to sports practices with the approval and under the supervision of their healthcare provider. When available, be sure to also work closely with your team's certified athletic trainer.

Below are five gradual steps that you, along with a healthcare provider, should follow to help safely return an athlete to play. Remember, this is a gradual process. These steps should not be completed in one day, but instead over days, weeks, or months.

Five-step Return To Play Progression

An athlete should only move to the next step if they do not have any new symptoms at the current step. If an athlete's concussion symptoms come back or if he or she gets new concussion symptoms, this is a sign that the athlete is pushing too hard. The athlete should stop these activities and the athlete's medical provider should be contacted. After more rest and no concussion symptoms, the athlete can start at the previous step.

Baseline: Back To School First

Athlete is back to their regular school activities, is no longer experiencing symptoms from the injury when doing normal activities, and has the green-light from their healthcare provider to begin the return to play process.

Step One: Light aerobic activity

Begin with light aerobic exercise only to increase an athlete's heart rate. This means about 5 to 10 minutes on an exercise bike, walking, or light jogging. No weight lifting at this point.

Step Two: Moderate activity

Continue with activities to increase an athlete's heart rate with body or head movement. This includes moderate jogging, brief running, moderate-intensity stationary biking, moderate-intensity weightlifting (less time and/or less weight from their typical routine).

Step Three: Heavy, noncontact activity

Add heavy noncontact physical activity, such as sprinting/running, high-intensity stationary biking, regular weightlifting routine, noncontact sport-specific drills (in 3 planes of movement).

Step Four: Practice and full contact

Young athlete may return to practice and full contact (if appropriate for the sport) in controlled practice.

Step Five: Competition

Young athlete may return to competition.

Chapter 38

Muscle Contusions (Bruises)

Produced by blunt trauma to the muscle, a muscle contusion or bruise is second only to strain as the leading type of injury that occurs in sports. A contusion can result from a simple fall or from the impact of jamming the body against a hard surface. Contusions do not involve a break in the skin. However, injury occurs to the soft tissues, including muscle fiber, blood vessels, or nerves. The injury typically shows up as a discoloration (ecchymoses) on the skin and is characterized by pain, tenderness, and swelling. The discoloration, caused by the pooling of blood from a ruptured blood vessel, starts off as a reddish-purple mark and changes color to blue-black, and eventually greenish-yellow as healing progresses. Muscle contusions are most common in contact sports such as football, boxing, and rugby.

Grading Of Muscle Contusions: Like sprains, contusions are graded depending on the severity:

- **Mild:** Caused by rupture of a small blood vessel, this is the least severe of contusions and is mostly asymptomatic. There is little or no pain and minimal loss of muscle function, and the individual can immediately return to his or her sport or activity.

- **Moderate:** Injury is slightly deeper than a mild contusion and involves pain, swelling, and a moderate loss of movement around the site of injury. Healing and return to activity after this type of injury usually takes anywhere between three and four weeks.

- **Severe:** This results from a massive blunt force to deep muscle tissues and is typically characterized by the formation of an intramuscular hematoma (a blood clot formed from a massive rupture of a blood vessel). When touched, the hematoma can be felt as a firm lump. This type of contusion is almost always accompanied by inflammation, intense pain, and complete loss of muscle function.

Diagnosis

Proper diagnosis of a contusion is an important factor in assessing the extent of injury and determining the line of treatment. A thorough clinical history of the trauma followed by a physical examination of the injured site is the first step in diagnosing soft tissue injuries. Sports medicine physicians also use imaging tests such as ultrasound, CT (computerized tomography), and MRI (magnetic resonance imaging) to assess any complications associated with the injury and to estimate recovery time.

Treatment

As with any type of soft tissue injury, the first line therapy for muscle contusion is the RICE (rest, ice, compression, and elevation) regimen. This treatment should be administered as soon as possible after the injury to reduce hemorrhage (bleeding), muscle spasms, and inflammation. Depending on the site and extent of injury, the elements of RICE therapy may be used together or as a combination of two or more elements.

- **Rest:** Conservative treatment of muscle contusion begins with immobilization of the injury site. A short period of early immobilization not only helps speedy repair of muscle tissues but also prevents chances of re-injury.

- **Ice:** The use of ice (also called cryotherapy) is effective in managing the acute phase (24–48 hours after injury) of a muscle contusion. Ice helps to reduce hemorrhage and thereby decreases the size of the hematoma. This, in turn, lowers inflammation and speeds up the regeneration of muscle tissue. Ice is usually applied for no longer than 15–20 minutes at a time.

- **Compression:** Wrapping the injured area with a bandage helps to reduce bleeding and edema (fluid buildup). Care should be taken to ensure a snug-fitting bandage. However, a wrapping that is too tight will cut off adequate blood flow to the injured muscle and cause more harm than good.

- **Elevation:** Raising the injured area to or above the level of your heart also helps to reduce pain and swelling by draining the excess fluid around the injured tissue back to the body's circulatory system.

Medication

Most contusions are treated with nonsteroidal anti-inflammatory drugs (NSAIDs). Analgesics (pain relievers) and muscle relaxants may also be prescribed to control pain and inflammation during the acute phase.

Rehabilitation

Proper rehabilitation is important to regain pain-free range of motion and restore normal muscle function. Any activity that puts stress on the injured area can compromise the healing process and negatively impact recovery. Rehabilitation should be supervised by sports therapists and begin with simple stretching exercises. This may be followed by strengthening and weight-bearing exercises for a few weeks before resuming normal activity.

Prognosis

While contusions are not considered serious injuries—as most tend to resolve on their own within a few weeks—the accompanying swelling and pain may cause discomfort and restrict movement. Deep muscle contusions may sometimes lead to complications that can have long-term effects and hamper recovery. One such complication is compartment syndrome. As the name suggests, this condition results from increased pressure in the muscle compartment, a confined space that encloses the muscle tissue, blood vessels, and nerves. Increased pressure in the muscle compartment is caused by rapid bleeding within the muscle tissue. This can cut off blood supply to the area, leading to extensive muscle and nerve damage. Surgery may be required to drain the excess fluids, release pressure, and prevent permanent muscle damage.

References

1. Crema, Michel D. "Imaging Techniques For Muscle Injury In Sports Medicine And Clinical Relevance," National Institute of Health (NIH), February 25, 2015.

2. Lazzaretti Fernandes, Tiago. "Muscle Injury—Physiopathology, Diagnosis, Treatment And Clinical Presentation," National Institute of Health (NIH), December 8, 2015.

3. Vorvick, Linda J. MD. "Bruise," National Institute of Health (NIH), April 11, 2017.

Chapter 39

Bursitis And Tendonitis

What Are Bursitis And Tendinitis?

Bursitis and tendinitis are both common conditions that cause swelling around muscles and bones. They occur most often in the shoulder, elbow, wrist, hip, knee, or ankle.

A bursa is a small, fluid-filled sac that acts as a cushion between a bone and other moving body parts such as muscles, tendons, or skin. Bursae are found throughout the body. Bursitis occurs when a bursa becomes swollen.

A tendon is a flexible band of tissue that connects muscles to bones. Tendons can be small, like those found in the hand or ankle, or large, like the Achilles tendon in the heel. Tendons help create movement by making the muscles push or pull the bones in different ways. Tendinitis is the severe swelling of a tendon.

What Causes These Conditions?

People get bursitis by overusing a joint. It can also be caused by direct trauma. It usually occurs at the knee or elbow. Kneeling or leaning your elbows on a hard surface for a long time can make bursitis start. Tendinitis usually occurs after repeated injury to a certain area such as the wrist or ankle. Tendons become less flexible with age and become more prone to damage.

Doing the same kinds of movements every day or putting stress on joints increases the risk for both conditions. People like carpenters, gardeners, musicians, and athletes often get bursitis or tendinitis. Infection, arthritis, gout, thyroid disease, and diabetes can also cause swelling of a bursa or tendon. Both bursitis and tendinitis are more frequent the older you get.

About This Chapter: This chapter includes text excerpted from "Bursitis—Fast Facts About Bursitis And Tendinitis," National Institute of Arthritis and Musculoskeletal and Skin Diseases (NIAMS), November 2014.

What Parts Of The Body Are Affected?

Tendinitis causes pain and soreness around a joint. Some common forms of tendinitis are named after the sports that increase their risk. They include tennis elbow, golfer's elbow, pitcher's shoulder, swimmer's shoulder, and jumper's knee.

Tennis Elbow And Golfer's Elbow

Tennis elbow is an injury to the tendon in the outer elbow. Golfer's elbow affects the inner tendon of the elbow. Any activity that involves a lot of wrist turning or hand gripping, such as using tools, shaking hands, or twisting, can bring on these conditions. Pain occurs near the elbow. It can also travel into the upper arm or forearm.

Shoulder Tendinitis, Bursitis, And Impingement Syndrome

Two types of tendinitis can affect the shoulder. Biceps tendinitis causes pain in the front or side of the shoulder. Pain may also travel down to the elbow and forearm. Raising your arm over your head may also be painful. The biceps muscle in the front of the upper arm helps secure the arm bone in the shoulder socket. It also helps control the speed of the arm during overhead movement. For example, you may feel pain when swinging a racquet or pitching a ball.

Rotator cuff tendinitis causes shoulder pain at the top of the shoulder and the upper arm. Reaching, pushing, pulling, or lifting the arm above shoulder level can make the pain worse.

Even lying on the painful side can worsen the problem. The rotator cuff is a group of muscles that attach the arm to the shoulder blade. This "cuff" allows the arm to lift and twist. Repeated motion of the arms can damage and wear down the tendons, muscles, and bone. Impingement syndrome is a squeezing of the rotator cuff.

Jobs that require frequent overhead reaching and sports involving lots of use of the shoulder may damage the rotator cuff or bursa. Rheumatoid arthritis also can inflame the rotator cuff and result in tendinitis and bursitis. Any of these can lead to severe swelling and impingement.

Knee Tendinitis Or Jumper's Knee

If you overuse a tendon during activities such as dancing, bicycling, or running, it may become stretched, torn, and swollen. Trying to break a fall can also damage tendons around the kneecap. This type of injury often happens to older people whose tendons may be weaker and less flexible. Pain in the tendons around the knee is sometimes called jumper's knee. This is because it often happens to young people who play sports like basketball. The overuse of the muscles and force of hitting the ground after a jump can strain the tendon. After repeated stress from jumping, the tendon may swell or tear.

People with tendinitis of the knee may feel pain while running, jumping, or walking quickly. Knee tendinitis can increase the risk for large tears to the tendon.

Achilles Tendinitis

The Achilles tendon connects the calf muscle to the back of the heel. Achilles tendinitis is a common injury that makes the tendon swell, stretch, or tear. It's usually caused by overuse. It can also result from tight or weak calf muscles. Normal aging and arthritis can also stiffen the tendon.

Achilles tendon injuries can happen when climbing stairs or otherwise overworking the calf muscle. But these injuries are most common in "weekend warriors" who don't exercise regularly or don't take time to warm up before they do. Among athletes, most Achilles injuries seem to occur in sprinting or jumping sports. Athletes who play football, tennis, and basketball can all be affected by Achilles tendinitis. An injury almost always retires the athlete for the rest of the season.

Achilles tendinitis can be a long-term condition. It can also cause what appears to be a sudden injury. When a tendon is weakened by age or overuse, trauma can cause it to rupture. These injuries can be sudden and agonizing.

How Are These Conditions Diagnosed?

Diagnosis of tendinitis and bursitis begins with a medical history and physical exam. You will describe the pain and when and where the pain occurs. The doctor may ask you whether it gets better or worse during the day. Another important clue is what makes the pain go away or come back. There are other tests a doctor may use including:

- Selective tissue tension test to find out which tendon is affected.

- Palpation or touching specific areas of the tendon to pinpoint the swelling.

- X-ray to rule out arthritis or bone problems.

- MRI (magnetic resonance imaging), which can show damage to both bone and soft tissue.

- Anesthetic injection test to see if the pain goes away.

- Taking fluid from the swollen area to rule out infection.

What Kind Of Healthcare Professional Treats These Conditions?

Your regular doctor or a physical therapist can treat most cases of tendinitis and bursitis. Cases that don't respond to normal treatment may be referred to a specialist.

How Are Bursitis And Tendinitis Treated?

The focus of treatment is to heal the injured bursa or tendon. The first step is to reduce pain and swelling. This can be done with rest, tightly wrapping or elevating the affected area, or taking drugs that bring down the swelling. Aspirin, naproxen, and ibuprofen all serve that purpose. Ice may be helpful in recent, severe injuries, but is of little or no use in long-term cases. When ice is needed, an ice pack can be held on the affected area for 15 to 20 minutes every 4 to 6 hours for 3 to 5 days. A healthcare provider may suggest longer use of ice and a stretching program.

Your healthcare provider may also suggest limiting activities that involve the affected joint.

Support equipment may be suggested such as:

- An elbow band for tennis elbow

- A brace for the ankle or foot

- A splint for the knee or hand

Other treatments may include:

- Ultrasound, which are gentle sound-wave vibrations that warm deep tissues and improve blood flow

- An electrical current that pushes a corticosteroid drug through the skin directly over the swollen bursa or tendon

- Gentle stretching and strengthening exercises

- Massage of the soft tissue.

If there is no improvement, your doctor may inject a drug into the area around the swollen bursa or tendon. If the joint still does not improve after 6 to 12 months, the doctor may perform surgery to repair damage and relieve pressure on the tendons and bursae.

If the bursitis is caused by an infection, the doctor will prescribe antibiotics.

If a tendon is completely torn, surgery may be needed to repair the damage.

Repairing a tendon tear requires an exercise program to restore the ability to bend and straighten the joint and to strengthen the muscles around it to prevent repeat injury. An exercise program may last 6 months.

Can Bursitis And Tendinitis Be Prevented?

To help prevent swelling or reduce the number of flares, you can do several things.

- Warm up or stretch before exercise.

- Strengthen the muscles around the joint.

- Take frequent breaks from repetitive tasks.

- Cushion the affected joint with foam (knee pads, elbow pads).

- Increase the gripping surface on tools by using gloves, grip tape, or other padding.

- Use an oversized grip on golf clubs.

- Use a two-handed backhand in tennis.

- Use two hands to hold heavy tools.

- Don't sit still for long periods.

- Practice good posture.

- Position your body properly when doing daily tasks.

- Begin new activities or exercises slowly.

- If you have a history of tendinitis, consider talking to your doctor before starting a new exercise.

Chapter 40

Facial Injuries

Broken Nose

The most common fracture that happens to the face, a broken nose, usually affects the bone over the bridge of the nose. A broken nose can result from a contact sport injury, fight, fall, or motor traffic accident. When you break your nose, you may experience severe pain, swelling, bruising, and bleeding from the nose. Your nose may appear crooked or misshapen, and you may face difficulty in breathing.

Complications

Complications of a broken nose may include:

- **Deviated septum.** Septum is the thin wall dividing the two sides of your nose. Nose fracture may cause the septum to be deviated. Surgery may be required to correct the condition.

- **Collection of blood.** Blood may collect inside the nose, blocking one or both nostrils. The collected blood may have to be drained by surgical means.

- **Neck injury.** A high-velocity injury to nose may also be accompanied by a neck injury—like those experienced in motor vehicle accidents.

Treatment

If the damage is not too serious, a broken nose can be treated with simple remedies such as:

- Act quickly. Start breathing through your mouth and lean forward to reduce the amount of blood that drains into your throat.

- Use ice packs or cold compresses immediately after the injury to help reduce swelling.

- Relieve pain by taking over-the-counter pain relievers like acetaminophen (Tylenol, others), ibuprofen (Advil, Motrin IB, others), or naproxen sodium (Aleve, others) as necessary.

- Keep your head up during sleep to prevent swelling and throbbing.

- Limit your activities by not playing in any sports at least for the first two weeks after treatment.

If the break is severe (the nose appears out of alignment or misshapen), a doctor may have to realign the bones. However, broken noses rarely require surgery.

Prevention

To prevent a fracture while playing sports, athletes should wear appropriate head gear and remain aware of their surroundings on the field or on the court.

Jaw Injuries

The jawbone, or mandible, is a U-shaped structure that extends from the chin to the ears. It connects to the skull at the temporomandibular joints (TMJ), which allow the jaw to open and close and move from side to side. Jaw injuries, such as a dislocated jaw or broken jaw (mandibular fracture), are fairly common in sports. The jawbone itself is vulnerable to fracture from impact with a ball or stick, while the TMJ can be damaged or unhinged from a blow to the mouth or a fall. Even athletes who take precautions like wearing a mouth guard and helmet can still experience jaw injuries because of the exposed location of the jawbone. Since jaw injuries can affect eating and breathing, they are considered serious conditions that require immediate medical attention.

Causes

Most jaw injuries occur due to facial trauma, such as a blow to the chin, mouth, or face. Although broken and dislocated jaws may occur due to motor vehicle accidents, industrial accidents, slip-and-fall accidents, or physical assaults, they are also common in sports. Sports that involve sticks—such as hockey, field hockey, and lacrosse—pose a particular risk of jaw injuries because of the additional force of swinging equipment. Fighting sports—such as boxing and mixed martial arts—also have a high incidence of jaw injuries. Yet broken and dislocated jaws can occur in many other types of sports and activities as well, including football, soccer, basketball, baseball, volleyball, skiing, and mountain biking.

Symptoms

When the mandible sustains a fracture, the bone typically breaks in multiple places on opposite sides of the jaw. A broken jawbone may remain in alignment, or it may be displaced or separated at the point of the fracture. In either case, the symptoms may include pain, swelling, bruising, bleeding from the mouth, loose teeth, and difficulty moving the jaw, speaking, or chewing. A displaced jaw fracture may involve additional symptoms, such as abnormality in the shape or appearance of the face, misalignment (malocclusion) of the teeth, and numbness in the chin and mouth. Symptoms of a dislocated jaw are likely to include pain, difficulty speaking and chewing, misalignment of the teeth, and drooling.

Diagnosis And Treatment

Jaw injuries should be considered medical emergencies. The immediate treatment—particularly if the athlete is unconscious—is to clear the airway of any broken teeth and blood. The athlete should then be positioned sitting up or lying on one side with their head tilted to allow any blood to run out of the mouth rather than into the throat. The jaw can be stabilized for transport to a hospital by gently wrapping gauze or an ace bandage under the chin and around the top of the head. An icepack can also be applied to help relieve pain and reduce swelling.

Diagnosis of a broken or dislocated jaw typically involves a physical examination and X-rays. Magnetic resonance imaging (MRI) or other tools may be used to determine whether muscles or ligaments in the face may be torn or damaged. Since jaw injuries most often result from a blow to the head, the athlete should also be evaluated for a possible concussion. Signs of concussion include headache, dizziness, confusion, nausea, ringing in the ears, sensitivity to light, and memory loss.

Treatment for a dislocated jaw involves returning it to the proper position through manual manipulation or surgery. A clean, minor, nondisplaced jaw fracture can often be immobilized and allowed to heal on its own. Severe, displaced, or multiple fractures of the jawbone, however, usually require surgical repair. In most cases, fractured or dislocated jaws must be wired together for four to six weeks to promote healing. A combination of wires and elastic bands are used to immobilize the jaw and align the teeth. Since the wires prevent the patient from opening their mouth, they cannot chew solid food and must obtain nutrition from a liquid diet. It is important to keep a wire-cutting tool on hand throughout the healing process in case the jaw must be opened due to choking or vomiting.

Recovery

Athletes who have an injury that requires their jaw to be wired shut must follow a liquid diet. Since they are unable to open their mouth or chew solid food, the available sources of nutrition are pureed fruits and vegetables, well-cooked meats, and soft grains taken through a straw. Experts recommend eating small, frequent meals and supplementing with whole milk, fruit juices, nutritional drinks, and even baby food to get enough calories and maintain weight. Even after the wires are removed, athletes should continue to follow a soft diet to protect the jaw during recovery. Pasta, rice, soup, canned meats, yogurt, and soft fruits are good choices, while raw produce, crunchy snacks, and chewy foods should be avoided.

Doctors usually approve light exercise—such as walking, resistance training, and stationery cycling—to maintain fitness and muscle tone while recovering from a jaw injury. If the jaw is wired, it is important to avoid strenuous exercise that requires breathing through the mouth. Most athletes can return to normal activities within a few months after the wires are removed. They may need to wear a mouth guard, face mask, or other protective device. Although broken and dislocated jaws heal successfully in most cases, some athletes experience recurring pain and stiffness in the jaw afterward—a condition known as temporomandibular joint disorder.

References

1. "Broken Nose," Mayo Clinic, June 18, 2014.

2. "Broken Nose (Nasal Fracture)—Topic Overview," WebMD, n.d.

3. "Be Smart About Jaw Injuries In Sports," MedCenter TMJ, February 16, 2016.

4. Roth, Erika. "Broken Or Dislocated Jaw," Healthline, 2015.

5. Ziegler, Terry. "Broken Jaw (Mandibular Fracture)," SportsMD, 2016.

Chapter 41

Eye Injuries

Sports Eye Injuries

Eye injuries are the leading cause of blindness in children in the United States and most injuries occurring in school-aged children are sports-related. These injuries account for an estimated 100,000 physician visits per year at a cost of more than $175 million.

Some sports carry a greater risk than others. For example, baseball is the leading cause of sports-related eye injury in children 14 and under and is considered high risk. Football carries a moderate risk. Check the table below for the risk categories for eye injury for various sports.

Eye Injuries: Sports That May Put You At Risk

Gear Up!

If you play sports, you know they can be a lot of fun. The last thing you want to do is miss a game, especially if it's because you're hurt. That's why you should always follow the rules and wear the right safety gear.

About This Chapter: Text under the heading "Sports Eye Injuries" is excerpted from "About Sports Eye Injury And Protective Eyewear," National Eye Institute (NEI), March 26, 2008. Reviewed July 2017; Text under the heading "Eye Injuries: Sports That May Put You At Risk" is excerpted from "Sports And Your Eyes," National Eye Institute (NEI), June 16, 2016; Text under the heading "Simple Steps To Prevent Eye Injuries In Sports" is excerpted from "Simple Steps To Prevent Eye Injuries In Sports," Office of Disease Prevention and Health Promotion (ODPHP), U.S. Department of Health and Human Services (HHS), October 1, 2014; Text under the heading "Protect Your Eyes When You Exercise" is excerpted from "Protect Your Eyes When You Exercise," Go4Life, National Institutes of Health (NIH), January 25, 2017; Text under the heading "First Aid Tips For Eye Injuries" is excerpted from "First Aid Tips," National Eye Institute (NEI), June 16, 2016.

Table 41.1. Sport-Specific Eye Injury Risk

High Risk	Moderate Risk	Low Risk
• Basketball	• Football	• Bicycling
• Boxing	• Golf	• Diving
• Hockey	• Badminton	• Skiing
• Paintball	• Soccer	• Swimming
• Racquetball	• Tennis	• Wrestling
• Softball	• Fishing	
• Squash		

Think about your favorite sport. Do you wear anything to protect your eyes, like goggles or a face mask? You might think you don't need protective eyewear, but sports-related eye injuries are serious. Eye injuries are a leading cause of blindness among children in the United States. The good news is that most eye injuries can be prevented with the right protective eyewear.

Protective Eyewear Fast Facts

- Everyone should wear protective eyewear.

- Ordinary prescription glasses, contact lenses, and sunglasses won't protect you from injuries. Most protective eyewear can be made to match your prescription.

- For the best protection, use eyewear made of ultra-strong polycarbonate.

- Choose eyewear specifically made for your sport and make sure it fits comfortably on your face.

Simple Steps To Prevent Eye Injuries In Sports

Most athletes think of knee and shoulder problems when we talk about sports-related injuries. With fall sports in full swing, it is important to remember that eye injuries in sports are not only common, but they are potentially very serious.

According to the American Academy of Ophthalmology (AAO), sports account for approximately 100,000 eye injuries each year. Roughly 42,000 of those injuries require evaluation in emergency departments. In fact, a patient with a sports-related eye injury presents to a United States emergency room every 13 minutes. It is estimated that sports-related eye injuries cost between $175 million and $200 million per year.

Generally baseball, basketball and racquet sports cause the highest numbers of eye injuries. One of every three of these eye injuries in sports occurs in children. In kids between the ages of five and 14, baseball is the leading cause. Basketball is a common culprit in athletes aged 15 and older. And boxing and martial arts present a high risk for serious eye injuries.

These eye injuries can be mild ones, but serious injuries like orbital fractures, corneal abrasions and detached retina can occur. Approximately 13,500 people become legally blind from sports-related eye injuries every year.

Fortunately the American Academy of Ophthalmology (AAO) estimates that 90 percent of eye injuries are preventable. October is Eye Injury Prevention Month, so athletes should remember these simple tips to avoid serious eye damage in sports:

- Wear appropriate eye protection, especially in basketball, racket sports, field hockey, and soccer. In baseball, ice hockey and men's lacrosse, an athlete should wear a helmet with a polycarbonate shield. Polycarbonate lenses are believed to be 10 times more resistant to impact than other materials. All protective eyewear should comply with American Society of Testing Materials (ASTM) standards.

- Wear additional protective eyewear, if you wear contact lenses or glasses. Contacts offer no protection against impacts to the eye. Glasses and sunglasses do not provide adequate protection and could shatter upon impact, increasing the danger to the eye.

- Wear eye protection for all sports if you are functionally one-eyed, meaning one eye has normal vision and the other is less than 20/40 vision

- Inspect protective eyewear regularly and replace when it appears worn or damaged.

Last, if an eye injury does occur, every athlete should consider going to an emergency department or consulting an ophthalmologist. Even a seemingly minor injury can actually be potentially serious and lead to loss of vision. Remember, 90 percent of sports-related eye injuries can be prevented.

Protect Your Eyes When You Exercise

Emergency room doctors treat an estimated 42,000 sports-related eye injuries each year in the United States. Nearly all of them could be prevented with protective eyewear.

Sports at moderate to high risk for eye injuries include: basketball, baseball, softball, ice hockey, tennis, soccer, volleyball, football, fishing, and golf. Studies show that protective eyewear does not hinder the player's sight while participating in athletics. In fact, some athletes can even play better because they're less afraid of getting hit in the eye.

Play it safe! Protect your eyes:

- Protective eyewear includes safety glasses and goggles, safety shields, and eye guards that are specially designed to provide the right protection for a certain activity.

- You still need protective eyewear that's approved for your sport even if you don't wear glasses or contacts.

- Ordinary prescription glasses, contact lenses, and sunglasses do not protect you from sports-related eye injury. You need to wear safety goggles over them.

- Experts recommend ultra-strong polycarbonate lenses for eye protection. Make sure they are in sport-appropriate frames or goggles.

- Many eye care providers sell protective eyewear, as do some sporting goods stores. Protective eyewear is sport-specific with the proper ASTM standards written on the packaging. This makes it easy to decide which pair is best for each activity.

First Aid Tips For Eye Injuries

Do you know what to do if you get sand in your eye? What if someone accidently elbows you in the eye during the game? Here are tips for dealing with some of the most common eye injuries. Remember to act fast and get help from an adult.

- If particles, like sand or dust, get into your eyes, don't rub! Wash your eyes out with water.

- If you get hit in the eye with a ball, rock, or elbow, gently put a cold compress on your eye for 15 minutes. This should make the swelling go down and relieve the pain. Have an adult take you to the doctor.

- If a chemical from a class experiment, cleaning fluid, or battery acid splashes in your eye, wash your eye out with water for at least 10 minutes. Have an adult take you to the doctor immediately.

- If an object like a stick or pencil gets stuck in your eye, don't pull it out. This is very serious. Have an adult put a loose bandage on your eye. Don't put any pressure on the object. Have an adult take you to the doctor immediately.

Chapter 42

Dental Injuries

While most people take care to wear appropriate padding, helmets, or other protective equipment when playing sports, roller skating, or bicycling, they often fail to take steps to guard against oral injuries.

While often overlooked, mouth guards are an important piece of athletic protective gear. Anyone who participates in organized sports or recreational activities is at risk for oral injuries, which can often require extensive and expensive corrective intervention. It is recommended that everyone from childhood to adulthood wear a mouth guard, even for noncontact sports.

What To Do In The Case Of Injury

Even with the use of safety equipment, dental injuries may occur. If an injury is severe enough to require a trip to the hospital emergency room, be sure to consult with an oral surgeon that has experience with your particular type of injury. An experienced oral surgeon may be able to detect hidden injuries that may not have been seen by emergency room personnel.

If a tooth was knocked loose or knocked completely out, it is important to act quickly. In some cases, the tooth can be saved. It is essential to immediately stop the activity, preserve the tooth, and go to a dentist immediately. However, time is of the essence as the tooth will begin to die after 15 minutes, and after two hours, the probability of saving the tooth is very low. There are some products available that are useful in preserving the tooth (e.g., as Save-A-Tooth). Your dentist can recommend other products you should include in your emergency first aid kit for treatment of mouth or tooth injuries.

About This Chapter: This chapter includes text excerpted from "OSHA Effective Ergonomics: Oral Sports Protection," Federal Occupational Health (FOH), U.S. Department of Health and Human Services (HHS), n.d. Reviewed July 2017.

If a permanent tooth is chipped or broken:

- Collect all the pieces of the tooth

- Rinse the damaged area of the mouth with warm water

- Use a cold compress to hold on the injured tooth

- See your dentist right away

If a permanent tooth is knocked out:

- Hold the tooth by the crown (the top), not the root.

- Rinse the tooth immediately with saline solution or milk. Tap water should be used only as a last resort; it contains chlorine, which may damage the root. Do not scrub the tooth.

- Keep the tooth from drying out. The best place to preserve the tooth on the way to the dentist is in its socket. Replace it gently, then bite down on a gauze pad to keep it in place. You can place the tooth under your tongue or between the cheek and gums. If this is impossible, store the tooth in milk (not water) or preserve it in a store bought tooth kit.

- See your dentist or go to an emergency room right away.

Selecting The Proper Oral Protection

According to the American Dental Association (ADA), there are three types of mouth guards. Mouth guards can be ready made, mouth formed, or custom-made. The most effective mouth guard is one that is made of a material that is resilient and tear-resistant. It should be light, fit properly, and be easy to clean. It is also important to consider the ease with which the athlete can breathe and speak while using this safety equipment. The guard should cover upper and or lower teeth and gums and be fitted so that it does not misalign the jaw and throw off the bite.

More elaborate protective equipment is recommended for high contact sports such as football, baseball, hockey, wrestling, boxing, and lacrosse. Some of these sports require additional safety devices such as chin straps, face guards, face masks, or helmets with wire cage face masks. It is best to consult your dentist for recommended safety gear that is specific to your sport(s), as well as unique dental needs.

Chapter 43

Spinal Cord Injuries

What Is Spinal Cord Injury (SCI)?

Spinal cord injury (SCI) is typically caused by a traumatic blow to (or penetration of) the spine that fractures or dislocates vertebrae. The trauma causes the resulting bone fragments, material in the spinal discs, or ligaments to bruise or tear into spinal cord tissue, damaging it or, in some cases, severing the cord entirely and resulting in partial or complete paralysis.

> - There are an estimated 12,000 spinal cord injuries every year in the United States alone.
> - More than a quarter of a million Americans are currently living with spinal cord injuries.
> - The cost of managing the care of spinal cord injury patients is $3 billion each year.
> - 80 percent of spinal cord injury patients are men.
>
> *(Source: "Spinal Cord Injury: Hope Through Research," National Institute of Neurological Disorders and Stroke (NINDS).)*

SCI is usually associated with what is commonly called a broken neck or broken back. Generally speaking, SCI is damage to the spinal nerves, the body's central and most important nerve bundle, as a result of trauma to the backbone.

Most cases of SCI take place when trauma breaks and squeezes the vertebrae, or the bones of the back. This, in turn, damages the axons—the long nerve cell "wires" that pass through

About This Chapter: This chapter includes text excerpted from "Spinal Cord Injury (SCI): Overview," *Eunice Kennedy Shriver* National Institute of Child Health and Human Development (NICHD), December 4, 2012. Reviewed July 2017.

vertebrae, carrying signals between the brain and the rest of the body. The axons might be crushed or completely severed by this damage. Someone with injury to only a few axons might be able to recover completely from their injury. On the other hand, a person with damage to all axons will most likely be paralyzed in the areas below the injury.

An SCI is described by its *level, type, and severity*. The *level* of injury for a person with SCI is the lowest point on the spinal cord below which sensory feeling and motor movement diminish or disappear.

The **level** is denoted by the letter-and-number name of the vertebra at the injury site (such as C3, T2, or L4).

- There are seven *cervical* vertebrae (C1 through C7), which are in the neck.

- There are 12 *thoracic* vertebrae (T1 through T12), which are located in the upper back. There are five *lumbar* vertebrae (L1 through L5), which are found in the lower back.

- Below those are five *sacral* vertebrae, which are fused to form the *sacrum*. Finally, there are the four vertebrae of the *coccyx*, or tailbone.

There are two broad **types** of SCI, each comprising a number of different levels:

- **Tetraplegia** (formerly called *quadriplegia*) generally describes the condition of a person with an SCI that is at a level anywhere from the C1 vertebra down to the T1. These individuals can experience a loss of sensation, function, or movement in their head, neck, shoulders, arms, hands, upper chest, pelvic organs, and legs.

- **Paraplegia** is the general term describing the condition of people who have lost feeling in or are not able to move the lower parts of their body. The body parts that may be affected are the chest, stomach, hips, legs, and feet. The state of an individual with an SCI level from the T2 vertebra to the S5 can usually be called paraplegic.

In addition, there are two degrees of SCI severity:

- **Complete injury** is the situation when the injury is so severe that almost all feeling (sensory function) and all ability to control movement (motor function) are lost below the area of the SCI.

- **Incomplete injury** occurs when there is some sensory or motor function below the damaged area on the spine. There are many degrees of incomplete injury.

The closer the spinal injury is to the skull, the more extensive is the curtailment of the body's ability to move and feel. If the lesion is low on the spine, say, in the sacral area, it is likely that there will be a lack of feeling and movement in the thighs and lower parts of the legs, the feet, most of the external genital organs, and the anal area. But the person will be able to breathe freely and move his head, neck, arms, and hands. By contrast, someone with a broken neck may be almost completely incapacitated, even to the extent of requiring breathing assistance.

What Are The Symptoms Of SCI?

According to the American Association of Neurological Surgeons (AANS), there are many different symptoms or signs of SCI. Some of the more common signs of SCI include:

- Extreme pain or pressure in the neck, head, or back

- Tingling or loss of sensation in the hand, fingers, feet, or toes

- Partial or complete loss of control over any part of the body

- Urinary or bowel urgency, incontinence, or retention

- Difficulty with balance and walking

- Abnormal band-like sensations in the thorax—pain, pressure

- Impaired breathing after injury

- Unusual lumps on the head or spine

What Causes SCI And How Does It Affect Your Body?

SCIs result from damage to the vertebrae, ligaments, or disks of the spinal column or to the spinal cord itself.

A traumatic SCI may stem from a sudden blow to the spine that fractures, dislocates, crushes, or compresses one or more vertebrae.

SCI has been caused by:

- Car crashes (40.4%)

- Falls (27.9%)

- Violence, including gunshot wounds (15%)

- Sport-related accidents (8%)

- Other/unknown (8.5%)

What Happens In Your Body When Your Spinal Cord Is Injured?

When an SCI occurs, the spinal cord starts to swell at the damaged area, cutting off the vital blood supply to the nerve tissue and starving it of oxygen. This sets off a cascade of devastation that affects the entire body, causing the injured spinal tissue to die, be stripped of its insulation, and be further damaged by a massive response of the immune system.

- Blood flow. The sluggish blood flow at the injury site begins to reduce the flow of blood in adjacent areas, which soon affects all areas of the body. The body begins to lose the ability to self-regulate, leading to drastic drops in blood pressure and heart rate.

- Flood of neurotransmitters. The SCI leads to an excessive release of neurotransmitters, or biochemicals that let nerve cells communicate with each other. These chemicals, especially glutamate, over excite nerve cells, killing them through a process known as excitotoxicity. The process also kills the vital oligodendrocytes that surround and protect the spinal axons with the myelin insulation that allows the spinal nerves to transmit information to and from the brain.

- Invasion of immune cells. An army of cells of the immune system speeds to the damaged area of the spine. While they help by preventing infection and cleaning up dead cellular debris, they also promote inflammation. These immune cells stimulate the release of certain cytokines that, in high concentrations, can be toxic to nerve cells, especially those needed to maintain the myelin sheath around axons.

- Onslaught of free radicals. The inflammation caused by cells in the immune system unleashes waves of free radicals, which are highly reactive forms of oxygen molecules. These free radicals react destructively with many types of cellular molecules, in the process severely damaging healthy nerve cells.

- Nerve cell self-destruction. A normally natural process of programmed cell death, known as apoptosis, goes out of control at the injury site. The reasons are not known. Days or weeks after the injury, oligodendrocytes die from no apparent cause, reducing the integrity of the spinal cord.

Additional damage usually occurs over the days or weeks following the initial injury because of bleeding, swelling, inflammation, and accumulation of fluid in and around the spinal cord.

How Is SCI Diagnosed?

SCIs are not always immediately recognizable. The following injuries should be assessed for possible damage to the spinal cord:

- Head injuries, particularly those with trauma to the face

- Pelvic fractures

- Penetrating injuries in the area of the spine

- Injuries from falling from heights

If any of these injuries occur together with any of the symptoms mentioned above (acute head, neck, or back pain; decline of feeling in the extremities; loss of control over part of the body; urinary or bowel problems; walking difficulty; pain or pressure bands in the chest area; difficulty breathing; head or spine lumps), then SCI may be implicated.

A person suspected of having an SCI must be carefully transported—to prevent further injury the spine should be kept immobile—to an emergency room or trauma center. A doctor will question the person to determine the nature of the accident, and the medical staff may test the patient for sensory function and movement. If the injured person complains of neck pain, is not fully awake, or has obvious signs of weakness or neurological injury, diagnostic tests will be performed.

These tests may include:

- CT ("CAT") scan

- MRI (magnetic resonance imaging) scan

- Myelogram

- Somatosensory evoked potential (SEP) testing or magnetic stimulation

- Spine X-rays

On about the third day after the injury, doctors give patients a complete neurological examination to diagnose the severity of the injury and predict the likely extent of recovery. This involves testing the patient's muscle strength and ability to sense light touch and a pinprick. Doctors use the standard ASIA (American Spinal Injury Association) Impairment Scale for this diagnosis. X-rays, MRIs, or more advanced imaging techniques are also used to visualize the entire length of the spine.

The ASIA Impairment Scale has five classification levels, ranging from complete loss of neural function in the affected area to completely normal:

- A: The impairment is complete. There is no motor or sensory function left below the level of injury.

- B: The impairment is incomplete. Sensory function, but not motor function, is preserved below the neurologic level (the first normal level above the level of injury) and some sensation is preserved in the sacral segments S4 and S5.

- C: The impairment is incomplete. Motor function is preserved below the neurologic level, but more than half of the key muscles below the neurologic level have a muscle grade less than 3 (i.e., they are not strong enough to move against gravity).

- D: The impairment is incomplete. Motor function is preserved below the neurologic level, and at least half of the key muscles below the neurologic level have a muscle grade of 3 or more (i.e., the joints can be moved against gravity).

- E: The patient's functions are normal. All motor and sensory functions are unhindered.

To illustrate, a person classified as C-level on the ASIA scale functions better than a person at the B level. Time was, a patient might have been labeled a C4 quadriplegic. Today, however, using the ASIA scale, the classification might be C4 ASIA A tetraplegic. Regarding muscle-strength grades, zero is the lowest, corresponding to complete absence of muscle movement. Five is the highest, representing full, normal strength.

What Are The Treatments For SCI?

Unfortunately, there are at present no known ways to reverse damage to the spinal cord. However, researchers are continually working on new treatments, including prostheses and medications, which may promote regeneration of nerve cells or improve the function of the nerves that remain after an SCI.

SCI treatment currently focuses on preventing further injury and empowering people with an SCI to return to an active and productive life.

At The Scene Of The Incident

Quick medical attention is critical to minimizing the effects of head, neck, or back trauma. Therefore, treatment for an SCI often begins at the scene of the injury.

Emergency personnel typically:

- Immobilize the spine as gently and quickly as possible using a rigid neck collar and a rigid carrying board

- Use the carrying board to transport the patient to the hospital

In The Emergency Room

Once the patient is at the hospital, healthcare providers focus on:

- Maintaining the person's ability to breathe

Recreation therapy encourages people with SCI to participate in recreational sports or activities at their level of mobility, as well as achieve a more balanced and normal lifestyle that provides opportunities for socialization and self-expression.

(Source: "Spinal Cord Injury: Hope Through Research," National Institute of Neurological Disorders and Stroke (NINDS).)

- Immobilizing the neck to prevent further spinal cord damage

Healthcare providers also may treat an acute injury with:

- Surgery

- Traction

- Methylprednisolone (Medrol)

- Experimental treatments

People with SCI may benefit from rehabilitation, including:

- Physical therapy geared toward muscle strengthening, communication, and mobility

- Use of assistive devices such as wheelchairs, walkers, and leg braces

- Use of adaptive devices for communication

- Occupational therapy focused on fine motor skills

- Techniques for self-grooming and bladder and bowel management

- Coping strategies for dealing with spasticity and pain

- Vocational therapy to help people get back to work with the use of assistive devices, if needed

- Recreational therapy such as sports and social activities

- Improved strategies for exercise and healthy diets (obesity and diabetes are potential risk factors for persons with SCI)

- Functional electrical stimulation for assistance with restoration of neuromuscular function, sensory function, or autonomic function (e.g., bladder, bowel, or respiratory function).

What Conditions Are Associated With SCI?

SCI is associated with many secondary conditions that have significant impacts on medical rehabilitation management, long-term outcome, and quality of life.

Secondary conditions associated with SCIs include:

- Breathing problems

- Bowel and bladder problems, including overactive bladder and incontinence

- Heart problems

- Pressure sores

- Sexual function problems

- Pain

- Blood clots

- Impaired muscle coordination (or spasticity)

- Pneumonia

- Autonomic dysreflexia (or hyperreflexia), which causes a potentially lethal increase in blood pressure

- Increased likelihood of certain cancers, including bladder cancer

Chapter 44

Shoulder Problems

What Are The Parts Of The Shoulder?

The shoulder joint is made up of bones held in place by muscles, tendons, and ligaments. Tendons are tough cords of tissue that hold the shoulder muscles to bones. They help the muscles move the shoulder. Ligaments hold the three shoulder bones to each other and help make the shoulder joint stable.

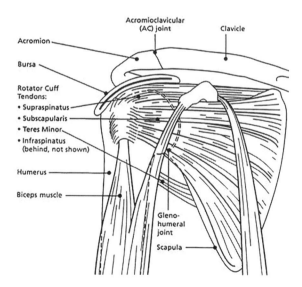

Figure 44.1. Structure Of The Shoulder

About This Chapter: This chapter includes text excerpted from "Fast Facts About Shoulder Problems," National Institute of Arthritis and Musculoskeletal and Skin Diseases (NIAMS), November 2014.

What Does It Mean?

Acromioclavicular (AC) joint: The joint of the shoulder located between the acromion (part of the scapula that forms the highest point of the shoulder) and the clavicle (collarbone).

Acromion: The part of the scapula (shoulder blade) that forms the highest point of the shoulder.

Arthrogram: A diagnostic test in which a contrast fluid is injected into the shoulder joint and an X-ray is taken to view the fluid's distribution in the joint. Leaking of fluid into an area where it does not belong may indicate a tear or opening.

Bursae: Filmy sac-like structures that permit smooth gliding between bone, muscle, and tendon. Two bursae cushion and protect the rotator cuff from the bony arch of the acromion.

Bursitis: Inflammation of the bursae that cushion joints. Bursitis is a common cause of shoulder pain.

Capsule: A soft tissue envelope that encircles the glenohumeral joint and is lined by a thin, smooth, synovial membrane.

Clavicle: The collarbone.

Corticosteroids: Powerful anti-inflammatory hormones made naturally in the body or manmade for use as medicine. Injections of corticosteroid drugs are sometimes used to treat inflammation in the shoulder.

Glenohumeral joint: The joint where the rounded upper portion of the humerus (upper arm bone) joins the glenoid (socket in the shoulder blade). This is commonly referred to as the shoulder joint.

Glenoid: The dish-shaped part of the outer edge of the scapula into which the top end of the humerus fits to form the glenohumeral shoulder joint.

Humerus: The upper arm bone.

Impingement syndrome: Squeezing of the rotator cuff, usually under the acromion.

Ligaments: Tough bands of connective tissue that attach bones to each other, providing stability.

Magnetic resonance imaging (MRI): A procedure in which a strong magnet is used to pass a force through the body to create a clear, detailed image of a cross section of the body. The procedure may be used to confirm the diagnosis of some shoulder problems.

Nonsteroidal anti-inflammatory drugs (NSAIDs): A class of medications that ease pain and inflammation and are available over the counter or with a prescription. Commonly used NSAIDs include ibuprofen (Advil, Motrin), naproxen sodium (Aleve), and ketoprofen (Actron, Orudis KT).

Osteoarthritis: The most common form of arthritis. It is characterized by the breakdown of joint cartilage, leading to pain, stiffness, and disability.

Rheumatoid arthritis: A form of arthritis in which the immune system attacks the tissues of the joints, leading to pain, inflammation, and eventually joint damage.

RICE: An acronym for rest, ice, compression, and elevation. These are four steps often recommended for treating musculoskeletal injuries.

Rotator cuff: Composed of tendons that work with associated muscles, this structure holds the ball at the top of the humerus in the glenoid socket and provides mobility and strength to the shoulder joint.

Scapula: The shoulder blade.

Synovial fluid: Lubricating fluid secreted by the synovial membrane that lines a joint.

Synovium: The membrane that lines the joint and secretes a lubricating liquid called synovial fluid.

Tendinitis: Inflammation of the tendons. In tendinitis of the shoulder, the rotator cuff and/or biceps tendon become inflamed, usually as a result of being pinched by surrounding structures.

Tendons: Tough cords of connective tissue that attach the shoulder muscles to bone and assist the muscles in moving the shoulder.

Transcutaneous electrical nerve stimulation (TENS): A technique that uses a small battery-operated unit to send electrical impulses to the nerves to block pain signals to the brain.

Who Gets Shoulder Problems?

Men, women, and children can have shoulder problems. They occur in people of all races and ethnic backgrounds.

What Causes Shoulder Problems?

Many shoulder problems are caused by the breakdown of soft tissues in the shoulder region. Using the shoulder too much can cause the soft tissue to break down faster as people get older. Doing manual labor and playing sports may cause shoulder problems.

Shoulder pain may be felt in one small spot, in a larger area, or down the arm. Pain that travels along nerves to the shoulder can be caused by diseases such as:

- Gallbladder disease

- Liver disease

- Heart disease

- Disease of the spine in the neck

249

> ## Shoulder Injury Among Young Athletes
>
> As participation in youth sports increases and younger children are playing a single sport year round, it is no wonder that more young athletes are being seen in doctors' offices in this country. For throwing sports like baseball and overhead sports like swimming and tennis, shoulder pain is a common complaint.
>
> **What Is Little League Shoulder (LLS)?**
>
> Little League shoulder (LLS) is an overuse injury to the proximal humerus (upper arm) originally described in young baseball players.
>
> **What Is The Treatment For LLS?**
>
> LLS does not require surgery. It does often involve a prolonged period of rest from throwing and overhead sports.
>
> *(Source: "Use Caution In Young Overhead Athletes With Shoulder Pain," Office of Disease Prevention and Health Promotion (ODPHP).)*

How Are Shoulder Problems Diagnosed?

Doctors diagnose shoulder problems by using:

- Medical history

- Physical examination

- Tests such as X-rays, ultrasound, and magnetic resonance imaging (MRI)

How Are Shoulder Problems Treated?

Shoulder problems are most often first treated with RICE (Rest, Ice, Compression, and Elevation):

- **Rest**. Don't use the shoulder for 48 hours.

- **Ice**. Put an ice pack on the injured area for 20 minutes, four to eight times per day. Use a cold pack, ice bag, or a plastic bag filled with crushed ice wrapped in a towel.

- **Compression**. Put even pressure (compression) on the painful area to help reduce the swelling. A wrap or bandage will help hold the shoulder in place.

- **Elevation**. Keep the injured area above the level of the heart. A pillow under the shoulder will help keep it up.

If pain and stiffness persist, see a doctor to diagnose and treat the problem.

What Are The Most Common Shoulder Problems?

The most common shoulder problems are:

- Dislocation

- Separation

- Rotator cuff disease

- Rotator cuff tear

- Frozen shoulder

- Fracture

- Arthritis

The symptoms and treatment of shoulder problems vary, depending on the type of problem.

Dislocation

Dislocation occurs when the ball at the top of the bone in the upper arm pops out of the socket. It can happen if the shoulder is twisted or pulled very hard.

To treat a dislocation, a doctor performs a procedure to push the ball of the upper arm back into the socket. Further treatment may include:

- Wearing a sling or device to keep the shoulder in place

- Rest

- Ice three or four times a day

- Exercise to improve range of motion, strengthen muscles, and prevent injury

Once a shoulder is dislocated, it may happen again. This is common in young, active people. If the dislocation injures tissues or nerves around the shoulder, surgery may be needed.

Separation

A shoulder separation occurs when the ligaments between the collarbone and the shoulder blade are torn. The injury is most often caused by a blow to the shoulder or by falling on an outstretched hand.

Treatment for a shoulder separation includes:

- Rest

- A sling to keep the shoulder in place

- Ice to relieve pain and swelling

- Exercise, after a time of rest

- Surgery if tears are severe

Rotator Cuff Disease: Tendinitis And Bursitis

In tendinitis of the shoulder, tendons become inflamed (red, sore, and swollen) from being pinched by parts around the shoulder.

Bursitis occurs when the bursa—a small fluid-filled sac that helps protect the shoulder joint—is inflamed. Bursitis is sometimes caused by disease, such as rheumatoid arthritis. It is also caused by playing sports that overuse the shoulder or by jobs with frequent overhead reaching.

Tendinitis and bursitis may occur alone or at the same time. Treatment for tendinitis and bursitis includes:

- Rest

- Ice

- Medicines such as aspirin and ibuprofen that reduce pain and swelling

- Ultrasound (gentle sound-wave vibrations) to warm deep tissues and improve blood flow

- Gentle stretching and exercises to build strength

- Injection of corticosteroid drug if the shoulder does not get better

- Surgery if the shoulder does not get better after 6 to 12 months

Rotator Cuff Tear

Rotator cuff tendons can become inflamed from frequent use or aging. Sometimes they are injured from a fall on an outstretched hand. Sports or jobs with repeated overhead motion can also damage the rotator cuff. Aging causes tendons to wear down, which can lead to a tear. Some tears are not painful, but others can be very painful.

Treatment for a torn rotator cuff depends on age, health, how severe the injury is, and how long the person has had the torn rotator cuff. Treatment for torn rotator cuff includes:

- Rest

- Heat or cold to the sore area

- Medicines that reduce pain and swelling

- Electrical stimulation of muscles and nerves

- Ultrasound

- Cortisone injection

- Exercise to improve range-of-motion, strength, and function

- Surgery if the tear does not improve with other treatments

Frozen Shoulder

Movement of the shoulder is very restricted in people with a frozen shoulder. Causes of frozen shoulder are:

- Lack of use due to chronic pain.

- Rheumatic disease that is getting worse.

- Bands of tissue that grow in the joint and restrict motion.

- Lack of the fluid that helps the shoulder joint move.

Treatment for frozen shoulder includes:

- Medicines to reduce pain and swelling

- Heat

- Gentle stretching exercise

- Electrical stimulation of muscles and nerves

- Cortisone injection

- Surgery if the shoulder does not improve with other treatments

Fracture

A fracture is a crack through part or all of a bone. In the shoulder, a fracture usually involves the collarbone or upper arm bone. Fractures are often caused by a fall or blow to the shoulder.

Treatment for a fracture may include:

- A doctor putting the bones into a position that will promote healing.

- A sling or other device to keep the bones in place.

- After the bone heals, exercise to strengthen the shoulder and restore movement.

- Surgery.

Arthritis Of The Shoulder

Arthritis can be one of two types:

1. Osteoarthritis—a disease caused by wear and tear of the cartilage.

2. Rheumatoid arthritis—an autoimmune disease causing one or more joints to become inflamed.

Osteoarthritis of the shoulder is often treated with nonsteroidal anti-inflammatory drugs (NSAIDs) such as aspirin and ibuprofen. People with rheumatoid arthritis may need physical therapy and medicine such as corticosteroids.

If these treatments for arthritis of the shoulder don't relieve pain or improve function, surgery may be needed.

Chapter 45

Arm Fractures

The human arm contains three long bones: the humerus, or upper arm bone, which extends from the shoulder to the elbow; and the radius and ulna, or forearm bones, which extend from the elbow to the wrist. The radius is located on the same side of the forearm as the thumb, while the ulna is located on the same side as the little finger. These two bones work together to rotate the forearm and turn the palm of the hand up or down. All three arm bones can be broken, or fractured, in the falls, collisions, and impacts that frequently occur in sports. The severity of arm fractures varies from minor cracks in the bone to open fractures in which displaced bone fragments penetrate through the skin. Less severe, nondisplaced arm fractures are usually treated conservatively, with immobilization in a cast, splint, or brace, while more severe fractures may require surgical repair.

Causes Of Arm Fractures

The most common type of arm fracture affects the forearm bones near the distal end, which is closest to the wrist. Forearm fractures also occur in the middle segment of the bones and near the proximal end, which is closest to the elbow. Fractures usually occur in both the radius and the ulna simultaneously, although either bone can also be broken independently. Forearm fractures are fairly common among young children who climb trees or jump off swings or other playground equipment. The injuries also occur frequently among active teens and adults who participate in sports, especially sports that involve physical contact or a risk of high-speed falls onto hard surfaces, such as skateboarding. Falling on an outstretched arm can break the radius or ulna, as can a direct blow to the forearm.

"Arm Fractures," © 2017 Omnigraphics. Reviewed July 2017.

Humerus fractures are less common than forearm fractures. They are typically caused by a direct impact to the upper arm in a high-speed collision or fall. A broken humerus can also result from falling on an outstretched arm or extreme twisting of the upper arm. A rare type of humerus fracture, known as a ball-thrower's fracture, happens when the upper arm muscles contract violently and create a spiral fracture around the bone. Outside of traumatic injuries, arm fractures sometimes occur in people whose bones are weakened by underlying medical conditions, such as osteoporosis or cancer.

Symptoms Of Arm Fractures

The symptoms of an arm fracture are similar regardless of which bone or bones have been broken. Depending on the severity of the fracture, the symptoms may include:

- pain
- swelling
- bruising
- limited range of motion
- visible deformity or shortening of the arm if the fracture is displaced
- numbness or weakness in the hand or wrist if nerves or blood vessels are injured
- bone fragments penetrating the skin in an open fracture

Diagnosis And Treatment For Arm Fractures

To diagnose an arm fracture, the doctor will review the athlete's medical history, including the circumstances under which the injury occurred and any previous history of injuries to the arm. Next, the doctor will evaluate the athlete's symptoms and conduct a medical examination of the arm, checking for areas of tenderness or deformity and testing range of motion, blood flow, and sensation. Finally, the doctor will order X-rays to confirm the diagnosis. X-rays can pinpoint the location of the fracture and show whether the bone is displaced or fragmented.

Humerus fractures can usually be treated without surgery. If there is mild displacement, the doctor may use a process called reduction to realign the parts of the bone. Then the athlete's arm will be immobilized in a cast, splint, or brace to protect it while the bone heals. Ice and anti-inflammatory medications can be used to relieve pain and reduce swelling. Once the fracture has healed, the athlete will need physical therapy or rehabilitation to restore strength and range of motion in the arm.

Since forearm fractures usually involve both the ulna and the radius, they are more likely to require surgery to maintain the proper rotating motion of the arm. Open fractures are almost always treated surgically due to the risk of infection from the bone puncturing the skin. Surgical treatment of an arm fracture involves aligning the pieces of the broken bone and stabilizing them to prevent movement while they heal. The surgeon will most likely use an internal fixation technique, which involves inserting metal plates and screws or a metal rod inside the arm to hold the bones together. Then the arm will be placed in a cast until the fractures heal. In the case of severe or multiple fractures, the surgeon may use an external fixation technique, which involves inserting metal pins or screws into the bone to hold a metal frame on the outside of the arm to stabilize the bone until it heals.

Recovery And Complications Of Arm Fractures

The recovery time for arm fractures depends on the severity of injury and type of treatment, as well as the patient's overall health. Minor fractures treated with a cast may only require four to eight weeks to heal, while severe fractures treated surgically may require twelve weeks or more. Although the prognosis for full recovery is very good for most arm fractures, it can take up to six months to regain full strength and range of motion in the arm.

Like all surgical procedures, surgery to repair arm fractures entails some risk of complications, including:

- infection

- damage to the surrounding nerves and blood vessels

- nonunion or malunion of the fracture, which may require additional surgery

- synostosis, a rare condition in which a bridge of bone forms between the radius and ulna during the healing process and limits range of motion in the forearm

References

1. "Adult Forearm Fractures," OrthoInfo, 2017.

2. "Arm Fracture," Drugs.com, 2017.

3. Imm, Nick. "Forearm Injuries And Fractures," Patient, 2014.

Chapter 46

Elbow Injuries

Tennis Elbow

Tennis elbow, or lateral epicondylitis, is an inflammation of the tendons that cause pain in the elbow and arm. The tendons involved are responsible for attaching the muscles that extend the wrist and hand. Tennis elbow produces pain on the outer part of the arm, unlike the similar condition called golfer's elbow, which affects the tendons on the inside of the elbow. Despite the name Tennis elbow, patients can have symptoms without ever stepping foot on a tennis court. Tennis elbow is the primary reason people see their doctor for elbow pain, and it is most commonly seen in the dominant arm. Although it can occur at any age, the most common age range is 30 to 50 years old, and affects an equal number of women and men.

What Causes Tennis Elbow?

Tennis elbow is considered a chronic condition because it occurs over time. Repetitive motions, such as using a screwdriver or swinging a racket, can put a strain on muscles and add stress to the tendons. The constant repetitive motion can eventually cause microscopic tears in the tissue surrounding the elbow. Tennis elbow can result from playing sports, but can also affect people with jobs or hobbies that require a recurring movement. A range of activities that involve repetitive motions include:

- **Sports:** Tennis, racquetball, fencing, golf

About This Chapter: Text under the heading "Tennis Elbow" is excerpted from "Tennis Elbow: Affecting More Than Just Tennis Players," National Aeronautics and Space Administration (NASA), July 19, 2007. Reviewed July 2017; Text under the heading "Osteochondritis Dissecans Of The Elbow (Little League Elbow)" is © 2017 Omnigraphics. Reviewed July 2017; Text under the heading "Ulnar Collateral Ligament Injuries (Thrower's Elbow)" is © 2017 Omnigraphics. Reviewed July 2017.

- **Work and Hobbies:** Typing, using a computer mouse, knitting, gardening, raking, using scissors, playing a musical instrument

- **Manual Occupations:** Painting, carpentry, plumbing, brick laying, using a screwdriver or hammer

What Are Common Symptoms Of Tennis Elbow?

Tennis elbow produces pain and tenderness on the lateral epicondyle, the bony knob on the outside of the elbow. The lateral epicondyle is where the inflamed tendons connect to the bone. In most cases the pain starts out mild and gradually becomes worse over weeks or months. Although the damage is in the elbow, there may be radiating or burning pain in the upper or lower arm, or outer part of the elbow. Pain may also occur when doing things with your hands. Tennis elbow may cause the most pain when:

- Lifting an object

- Gripping an object or making a fist

- Extending the forearm or straightening the wrist

- Shaking hands or opening a door

- Pressing on the outer surface of the elbow

To properly diagnose tennis elbow, your athletic trainer or doctor will do a thorough examination. The athletic trainer or doctor may have you flex your arm, wrist, and elbow to see where it hurts, and may press on the lateral epicondyle to reproduce symptoms. In more severe cases you may also need an X-ray or MRI (magnetic resonance imaging) to detect tennis elbow or rule out other problems.

What Are Treatment Options For Tennis Elbow?

Tennis elbow will usually heal on its own if you rest the injured tendon by stopping or changing your activity. If pain increases or the condition continues and is left untreated, a loss of function may occur so it is important to seek medical care. Types of helpful treatment are:

- **Reduce inflammation and pain:** Rest, ice, elevation, and compression (RICE), Non-steroidal anti-inflammatory drugs (NSAIDs), such as ibuprofen according to package directions, injections of steroids or painkillers to temporarily relieve symptoms

- **Rehabilitation:** Perform range of motion exercises to decrease stiffness and increase flexibility, physical therapy to strengthen the muscles

- **Orthotics:** An elbow strap or wrist splint to restrict the movement of the tendon and protect from further strain

- **Activity Modification:** Improve posture and technique, alternate hands during activities, use a smaller grip on tools or rackets, have a workstation assessment

Nonoperative treatment is successful in about 90 percent of patients with tennis elbow, but in severe cases with symptoms lasting 4–6 months, surgery may be required. The outpatient procedure consists of removing the section of the damaged tendon and repairing the remaining tendon. Surgery is only required in a small amount of patients seen with Tennis elbow, and the success rate of the procedure is very high.

When Can I Return To Normal Activities?

Returning to regular activities depends on the individual case and extent of the damage to the tendon. People heal at different rates so it is important to not rush recovery and to not push yourself. Although there may be a period of relief, pain may come back, and ending a treatment plan early may increase the chance of reinjury. You may be able to start performing normal levels of activity if:

- The injured elbow is no longer swollen

- The injured elbow feels as strong as the noninjured elbow

- The elbow can be flexed with no trouble

- Bearing weight is no longer painful

- You can grip objects pain-free

How Can I Prevent Tennis Elbow?

The best way to prevent Tennis elbow is to avoid overuse. If any pain is felt during activity you should stop and rest the elbow. If symptoms arise during activities at work, frequent breaks should be taken.

Tennis elbow can develop from using the wrong equipment, such as a racket that is too heavy, or a golf club that has a grip that is too large. Poor posture and bad technique may also lead to Tennis elbow. To help prevent Tennis elbow it is important to:

- Stretch and warm up before using the upper extremities

- Ice the elbow after activity

- Use alternate hands during activities to prevent overuse

- Strengthen the muscles of the arm, elbow, wrist, and back

- Use correct technique

Osteochondritis Dissecans Of The Elbow (Little League Elbow)

Osteochondritis dissecans (OCD) is an overuse injury that involves damage and deterioration of the articular cartilage that cushions and protects the elbow joint. Ongoing, forceful use of the arm disrupts the blood supply to the cartilage and the underlying subchondral bone, which eventually causes small pieces of cartilage and bone to weaken, crack, break off, and interfere with the function of the elbow joint. OCD is sometimes referred to as Little League elbow because the injury has been associated with the repetitive stress of pitching a baseball, but it also affects young people who play other sports that place strain on the elbow, such as gymnastics, tennis, and weightlifting. OCD usually affects people between the ages of 10 and 20 whose bones are still growing and thus are more prone to injury. In contrast, adult elbow injuries typically affect ligaments and tendons rather than bones.

Causes And Symptoms

Since OCD of the elbow often affects several members or generations of the same family, some experts believe that the condition has a genetic component that makes some people more likely to develop it. Research also suggests that overuse strain contributes to the development of the condition. Most adolescents who are treated for OCD of the elbow are active in sports that involve repeated, forceful throwing, hitting, pulling, or landing actions that place stress on the elbow joint, causing the bones to jam into the articular cartilage over and over again. Since the cartilage is immature and the bones are still growing, the repeated impacts can cause damage to the elbow joint.

The symptoms of elbow OCD typically appear gradually and worsen over time. In fact, 80 percent of athletes diagnosed with the condition cannot recall a specific injury to their elbow. The first sign of a problem is usually pain or discomfort while engaging in the activity that is creating repetitive stress on the elbow joint. As the condition worsens, athletes may experience the following additional symptoms:

- aching of the elbow while not playing sports

- sharp pain when bending or straightening the arm

- swelling on the inside of the elbow joint

- stiffness and difficulty straightening the elbow

- grinding, crackling, or popping sounds (crepitus) when moving the elbow joint

- catching or locking of the elbow as loose cartilage or bone chips interfere with joint function.

Diagnosis

To make a diagnosis of OCD of the elbow, the doctor will take a medical history and conduct a physical examination. The doctor will inquire about the athlete's age and involvement in sports and activities that cause repetitive stress to the elbow joint, such as baseball, tennis, and gymnastics. The doctor will then examine the sore elbow for swelling and tenderness and compare it to the healthy elbow. Next, the doctor will evaluate the range of motion in each elbow and check for crepitus during elbow movement.

The doctor will order diagnostic imaging tests to help determine the condition of the bones and cartilage in the elbow joint. Although X-rays of athletes with elbow OCD sometimes appear normal, they may show irregularities in the elbow joint, such as changes in shape, size, or alignment. X-rays can also show whether the athlete's growth plates remain open and detect the presence of cracks or bone chips. Magnetic resonance imaging (MRI) or computed tomography (CT) scans may also be used to get a more accurate picture of the bones and tissues in the elbow joint, as well as to monitor changes during the healing process.

Treatment

Treatment of elbow OCD depends on the severity of the condition. Most experts prefer to treat mild cases conservatively, with a combination of rest, bracing, and physical therapy. Younger athletes and those with early cartilage damage that has not progressed to the point of deterioration and tearing are the best candidates for this approach. The athletes are advised to stop engaging in the repetitive action that caused the elbow soreness for around six weeks, although they are usually encouraged to continue exercising to maintain fitness. A baseball pitcher, for instance, might be able to serve as designated hitter or play a position that does not demand much throwing, like first base. Conservative care may also include prescription or over-the-counter anti-inflammatory medications to help relieve pain and swelling, as well as regular application of ice to the elbow. Some experts recommend wearing a hinged brace to support the elbow during the rest period as well as when the athlete resumes activities.

Following a period of complete rest of the affected elbow, athletes must undergo physical therapy to strengthen and stretch muscles and regain range of motion in the joint. A key part of physical therapy for elbow OCD involves activity modification, in which athletes learn methods of changing their body mechanics to improve form and reduce strain on to the elbow. When pain and other symptoms disappear, athletes can make a slow, gradual return to competition. Baseball pitchers, for example, should follow a strict program that gradually increases the number, distance, and effort of throws. Although many young athletes will be tempted to return to action quickly, failure to follow the treatment plan can lead to serious, lifelong elbow conditions like arthritis.

For more severe cases of elbow OCD, the treatment is likely to involve surgery. This approach is often necessary for athletes who continue to experience symptoms after completing six months of conservative treatment, as well as for those who have fragments of cartilage and bone—known as loose bodies—restricting movement of the elbow joint. Procedures used to treat OCD of the elbow may be performed as open surgery through an incision on the outer part of the elbow, or as minimally invasive arthroscopic surgery using an instrument with a tiny camera mounted on the end. The most commonly used surgical techniques include the following:

- **Drilling**

  For elbow OCD that has not yet produced loose bodies, the surgeon may use a special instrument to drill tiny holes through the damaged articular cartilage and into the healthy layer of bone underneath. Drilling stimulates a healing response in the bone marrow, causing drops of blood to fill the holes and new cartilage to grow in the damaged area.

- **Debridement**

  This method is generally used when cartilage and bone in the elbow joint is damaged or torn, but remains attached. The surgeon uses a small instrument to shave away (debride) irritated, loose, or dead tissue from the joint. The surface of the bone is smoothed down until it bleeds, which stimulates the bone marrow to fill in the damaged area.

- **Pinning**

  When advanced OCD has caused pieces of bone or cartilage to detach from the elbow joint, the surgeon may debride the damaged area and then use surgical wires to pin the fragments back in place.

- **Grafting**

  In some cases, the surgeon may attempt to repair an area of damaged articular cartilage in the elbow by replacing it with a graft of tissue transplanted from a different joint. The osteochondral autograft transplantation (OAT) technique involves harvesting healthy plugs of bone and cartilage, usually from the knee joint, and transferring them to the elbow. However, differences between knee and elbow cartilage can make it challenging to match the graft with the shape of the damaged area.

Recovery And Prevention

Although surgery can relieve pain, provide stability, and increase range of motion in the elbow, few athletes are able to regain peak form afterward. Most young athletes with elbow OCD that is severe enough to require surgery are forced to modify their activities or stop playing high-level sports. The main goal of surgical treatment is to prevent the development of degenerative arthritis in the elbow in adulthood.

Fortunately, there are ways to prevent the development of elbow OCD in young athletes, including the following:

- pay close attention to symptoms and cease activities that cause elbow pain until symptoms subside

- limit pitch counts for young baseball players, and avoid throwing breaking pitches—which cause the most elbow stress—until age 14 for a curveball and 16 for a slider

- avoid specialization in a single sport year-round, and promote cross-training in multiple sports

- emphasize the benefits of resistance training, conditioning, and physical fitness

- teach proper mechanics and form to reduce the risk of injury.

Ulnar Collateral Ligament Injuries (Thrower's Elbow)

The ulnar collateral ligament (UCL) is a thick, triangular band of connective tissue on the inside of the elbow that links the humerus (upper arm bone) to the ulna (forearm bone on the same side as the pinkie finger). The UCL plays an important role in stabilizing the elbow joint, particularly during overhead motions like throwing a ball. The ligament can become stretched, damaged, or torn from overuse in the repeated, forceful overhead motions that are commonly performed in such sports as baseball, football, volleyball, water polo, cricket, and tennis. As a result, the injury is sometimes called "thrower's elbow." Although minor UCL injuries can heal on their own, surgery is sometimes required to repair tears in the ligament and restore stability to the elbow joint. The UCL reconstruction procedure is often referred to as "Tommy John surgery" after the famous Major League Baseball pitcher who became the first person to undergo it in 1974.

Causes

Repetitive stress from forceful throwing motions is the most common cause of ulnar collateral ligament injuries. Athletes like professional pitchers who throw hard on a regular basis place a great deal of strain on the UCL, causing tiny tears to develop in the soft tissue. These microtears accumulate over time, causing weakness and degeneration of the ligament. Eventually, the UCL may tear, rupture, or "pop," resulting in pain and instability in the elbow joint. Other contributing factors to thrower's elbow may include failure to warm up and cool down properly, poor throwing mechanics or technique, lack of rest between throwing sessions, and use of improper or ill-fitting equipment. In addition to overuse, UCL tears can also be caused by an acute injury, such as falling onto an outstretched hand.

A related condition that develops in adolescents between the ages of 10 and 20 is known as Little League elbow. Since the bones of young athletes are still growing, the type of repetitive throwing motions that place stress on the UCL typically damage the growth plate in the elbow rather than the ligament itself. In advanced cases, pieces of cartilage and bone break off and interfere with movement of the elbow joint.

Symptoms And Diagnosis

Pain in the elbow when throwing is the first sign of injury to the UCL. The pain may radiate down the forearm into the wrist or hand, and the inside of the elbow may feel tender or appear slightly swollen. If condition progresses to the point where the ligament ruptures, many athletes report hearing a popping sound, which is immediately followed by pain, weakness, and instability in the elbow joint. Finally, some athletes also experience numbness or tingling in the forearm and hand.

To diagnose a UCL injury, a doctor will begin by taking a health history, which will include questions about the athlete's participation in sports and the onset and duration of symptoms. Next, the doctor will conduct a physical examination of the elbow, manipulating it gently to identify the source of pain. One test of elbow strength and stability is the valgus stress test, in which the doctor applies pressure to the outside of the elbow joint while bending the arm. The doctor will also order diagnostic imaging tests, such as magnetic resonance imaging (MRI) or magnetic resonance arthrogram (MRA), to view areas of damage in the elbow joint.

Treatment

Treatment for the early stages of UCL injury is usually conservative. At the onset of symptoms, the athlete may be advised to rest the elbow for several days, apply ice to the area, take anti-inflammatory medications, and wear an elbow brace or compression sleeve. Once the pain has gone away, the athlete may be urged to perform physical therapy or rehabilitation to improve the strength, flexibility, stability, and range of motion of the elbow joint.

For severe cases, in which the UCL has ruptured, treatment involves surgical reconstruction of the ligament. The surgeon makes an incision on the inside of the elbow, splits and retracts the flexor muscles to reveal the UCL beneath, and replaces the damaged ligament with a tendon taken from the athlete's arm, leg, or foot.

There are two main surgical techniques used to replace the UCL ligament. In the docking technique, the surgeon drills two holes in the ulna and three holes in the medial epicondyle at the end of the humerus. The new tendon is looped through the holes in the ulna, stretched across the elbow joint, and threaded through the bottom hole in the medial epicondyle. Next, sutures attached to the ends of the tendon are passed through the upper holes in the medial epicondyle. The surgeon uses these sutures to pull the tendon tight and adjust its tension to allow a full range of movement in the elbow. When the optimal tension has been achieved, the surgeon ties off the sutures.

In the figure of eight technique, the surgeon drills two holes in the ulna and two holes in the medial epicondyle. The new tendon graft is looped through all four holes in a figure-eight pattern and then sutured together. After surgery, the athlete's elbow is bandaged and placed in a splint for several weeks to protect it while it heals. Although rehabilitation from Tommy John surgery can take more than a year, more than 80 percent of pitchers who undergo it are able to return to their previous level of competition.

Prevention

The key to preventing UCL injuries is to avoid overuse and repetitive stress of the elbow. Experts recommend taking the following precautions to protect the UCL from damage:

- warm up and stretch before any throwing activity

- perform regular strength and conditioning of the arms, shoulders, and core

- cool down properly following activity

- limit pitch counts and allow recovery time between games

- avoid playing a single sport year round

- pay attention to proper body and throwing mechanics

- cease throwing immediately upon experiencing pain

- seek medical treatment if pain persists following rest, ice, and anti-inflammatory medication.

References

1. Dikmanis, Andris. "Fitness And Training: Thrower's Elbow," *Baseball Player Magazine,* July 1, 2010.

2. "Physical Therapist's Guide To Ulnar Collatoral Ligament Injury," Move Forward PT, 2017.

3. Walker, Brad. "Throwers Elbow And Throwers Elbow Treatment," Stretch Coach, 2017.

4. "Adolescent Osteochondritis Dissecans Of The Elbow," Orthopod, n.d.

5. "Little League Elbow," Healthy Children, November 21, 2015.

6. "Preferred Treatment For OCD Of The Elbow," Active Sport Physiotherapy Clinic, 2014.

7. Savoie III, Felix H. "Osteochondritis Dissecans Of The Elbow," *Operative Techniques in Sports Medicine,* 2008.

Chapter 47

Wrist Fractures

The wrist is made up of ten separate bones: the two bones of forearm (called radius and ulna) and eight small bones at the base of the hand. A wrist fracture can happen in any of these ten bones. However, the most common fracture is the distal radius fracture, or Colles fracture, that occurs at the lower end of the radius. The Irish surgeon and anatomist, Abraham Colles, described this fracture in 1814 and hence the name "Colles" fracture.

Studies show that 1 out of every 10 broken bones is a broken wrist in the United States. This type of fracture commonly occur in contact sports, skiing, skating, and biking and the usual cause of injury is the athlete throwing out his or her hand to break a fall, known as a Fall on an Outstretched Hand (FOOSH) injury.

The break in the distal radius fracture can be of various types, such as:

- Nondisplaced stable fracture, meaning that the bone has broken but the pieces have remained in place.

- A break in lower end of the radius that can extend into the wrist joint.

- A piece of broken bone that breaks through the skin (an open fracture).

- The bone may shatter into many pieces, known as a comminuted fracture.

- Unstable fractures with larger broken fragments that are not in place.

The above classification of a fracture is important because the course of treatment and the outcome is based on the nature of the fracture. Open and comminuted fractures are difficult to treat and residual problems like stiffness and deformity can result.

"Wrist Fractures," © 2017 Omnigraphics. Reviewed July 2017.

Causes Of Wrist Fractures

FOOSH is the most common cause for wrist fractures. Osteoporosis, a condition in which bone become weak and porous, is another common cause, where even minor falls can result in a broken wrist. Severe trauma such as road traffic accidents and contact sports injuries can also cause bad fractures of the wrist.

Signs And Symptoms Of Wrist Fractures

- Pain and swelling around the wrist.

- Difficulty moving and using the wrist and hand.

- Deformity—the wrist hangs or bends unnaturally.

- Tingling sensation or numbness in the fingers.

Diagnosis Of Wrist Fractures

The surgeon will perform a physical examination of the wrist and hand. A set of X-rays will be ordered to ascertain the nature and location of the fracture. If the fracture is complicated, a computed tomography (CT) or magnetic resonance imaging (MRI) scan would be needed to get better details of the fracture fragments and soft tissue (ligaments) damages around the fracture.

Treatment For Wrist Fractures

Fractures are treated either by surgical or nonsurgical methods depending on the nature of the fracture.

If the fractured segments are stable and in good position nonsurgical treatment methods can be used.

If there is a displacement, realignment of the fractured segments are done by a surgeon and plaster cast will be applied. This is usually done under sedation by applying traction force on the fractured segments. This method is called closed reduction. There will be a repeat plaster casting 2 to 3 days later after the swelling subsides. Check X-rays will be taken during this period to make sure the fractured segments are in position.

A fracture with multiple displaced fragments and punctured skin makes it an unstable open fracture. This will require surgery for proper fracture reduction and immobilization. This surgical method is called open reduction and internal fixation (ORIF) where metal pins, wires, plates and screws are used to fix the fractures.

One basic rule common to both surgical and nonsurgical methods is putting the fractured segments back in position with proper alignment and preventing it from moving out of place. This is to prevent deformity and ensure full range of movements in the joints and return to normal functional activities.

The treatment method also depends on various other factors of the person such as their age, nature of sport, level of activity, and their overall health.

Recovery From Wrist Fractures

Pain: After a wrist fracture, a patient will experience a considerable amount of pain for a few days or weeks. Ice, elevation of the hand, and nonsteroidal anti-inflammatory drugs (NSAIDs) will help in coping with pain.

Cast care: Make sure you keep the cast dry. If it loosens as the swelling comes down, it has to be reapplied. If you have unrelenting pain, it is a warning sign for you to contact your surgeon.

It is important to keep moving your fingers, elbow and shoulder to prevent them from getting stiff.

Return To Play

Once the cast is removed, your physical therapist will work on your wrist and hand to get back the range of movement and functional ability. You will be able to resume lighter activities like swimming or exercising the lower body by 1 or 2 months after removing of the cast. Vigorous sports activities can be resumed after 3 to 6 months.

References

1. "Wrist Fractures," American Society for Surgery of the Hand (ASSH), 2015.

2. "Distal Radius Fractures (Broken Wrist)," American Academy of Orthopaedic Surgeons (AAOS), 2013.

3. "Colles' Fracture (Distal Radius Fracture Or Broken Wrist)," WebMD, 2017.

4. "Wrist Fractures," Patient Platform Limited, 2016.

Chapter 48

Groin Injuries

Sportsman's Hernia

Chronic groin pain is a frequent cause for referral to general surgeons. In some cases this pain may be due to the presence of a hernia. However, if on clinical examination there is no palpable lump or bulge, the cause of the pain may be difficult to elucidate. Some of these patients may have the diagnosis of sportsman's groin. Other names which have been attached to this condition include Gilmore groin and sportsman's hernia. These conditions are more commonly associated with sportsmen and women but those who do not play sport may also receive this diagnosis. Sportsman's groin is thought to be a syndrome of weakness of the posterior inguinal wall without a clinically recognizable hernia. Differing explanations for sportsman's groin include avulsion of the conjoint tendon from the pubic tubercle, weakening of the transversalis fascia, tears in the internal or external oblique, superficial inguinal ring dilatation and abnormalities of the rectus abdominus insertion.

About This Chapter: Text under the heading "Sportsman's Hernia" is excerpted from "A Randomised, Blinded Study On Laparoscopic Mesh Reinforcement For Chronic Groin Pain," ClinicalTrials.gov, National Institutes of Health (NIH), March 15, 2010. Reviewed July 2017; Text beginning with the heading "Symptoms And Diagnosis" is excerpted from "TEP Versus Open Minimal Suture Repair For The Sportsman's Groin (SPORT)," ClinicalTrials.gov, National Institutes of Health (NIH), November 19, 2014; Text beginning with the heading "Perineal Injury In Males" is excerpted from "Perineal Injury In Males," National Institute of Diabetes and Digestive and Kidney Diseases (NIDDK), March 2014; Text under the heading "Using No-Nose (Noseless) Bicycle Saddles To Prevent Genital Numbness And Sexual Dysfunction" is excerpted from "Using No-Nose (Noseless) Bicycle Saddles To Prevent Genital Numbness And Sexual Dysfunction," Centers for Disease Control and Prevention (CDC), March 2, 2017.

Symptoms And Diagnosis

The prevalence of chronic groin pain in athletes and physically active adults is between 5 and 10 percent. The groin area is vulnerable in contact sports such as soccer, ice hockey, and rugby that require sudden muscle contraction around the hip and lower abdomen, repetitive kicking and side-to-side motion. Common causes for chronic groin pain in such sports include adductor tendonitis, musculus rectus abdominis tendopathy, osteitis pubis or disruption of the posterior wall of inguinal canal, which are all referred to as athletic pubalgia. No exact pathophysiological mechanism for pain has so far been identified in sportsman's hernia (posterior inguinal wall deficiency). A tear of the abdominal wall in posterior inguinal canal or conjoined tendon (tendinopathy), with or without bulging of a hernia, is suggested to be typical of a sportsman's hernia. The tissue damage is similar as in an incipient direct inguinal hernia with or without bulge.

Diagnosis of a sportsman's hernia can only be set in patients having a typical history and having a suspected posterior inguinal wall deficiency on careful clinical examination. Magnetic resonance imaging (MRI) should be performed to exclude other injuries in the groin area. Sometimes ultrasonography would be added in the diagnostic work-up. Although presenting with similar symptoms, the clinical entity of "sportsman's hernia" is exclusively distinct from athletic pubalgia, which includes a more wide range of groin injuries, such as adductor tendonitis and/or inflammation of the pubic symphysis.

Treatment

Treatment of chronic groin pain is aimed toward its specific pathology. The first line of management includes rest, muscle strengthening and stretching exercises, physiotherapy, anti-inflammatory analgesics, as well as local anesthetic and/or corticosteroid injections. In resistant cases, operative treatment might be considered. Various operative approaches in athlete's pubalgia have been proposed depending on the suspected nature of injury. These operative approaches include open and laparoscopic methods of hernia repair, tenotomy of muscle tendons close to the pubic bone, as well as release or neurectomies of nearby nerves. The results of operative treatment are good to excellent in 70 to 90 percent of patients. There is no evidence-based consensus available to guide surgeons for choosing between various operative treatments of sportsman's hernia/athletic pubalgia. Both conventional open and laparoscopic repairs produce good results, although the latter may allow the patient to an earlier return to full sports activity.

Open minimal repair (OMR) technique in local or spinal anesthesia seems to be a promising surgical approach in the treatment of posterior inguinal wall deficiency. This is best described as open minimal repair and involves a small incision into the groin of the affected side. Once the inguinal canal is exposed the back wall is repaired using a simple suture to reinforce the weakness. An one-center analysis of this technique reported full freedom of pain in 91 percent four weeks after operation, full recovery to sports after 2 weeks and good patient's satisfaction in 100 percent. The laparoscopic techniques are reported to give an excellent outcome in 80–90 percent of patients. These methods are more expensive and need to be performed under general anesthesia. The OMR technique is developed solely to strengthen the posterior inguinal wall weakness using nonabsorbable sutures. Endoscopic total extraperitoneal (TEP) technique in general anesthesia is also used for the treatment of Sportsman's hernia/athletic pubalgia and may heal a wider area in groin. TEP utilizes a mesh placed in the preperitoneal space behind the pubic symphysis and posterior inguinal canal.

Perineal Injury In Males

Perineal injury is an injury to the perineum, the part of the body between the anus and the genitals, or sex organs. In males, the perineum is the area between the anus and the scrotum, the external pouch of skin that holds the testicles. Injuries to the perineum can happen suddenly, as in an accident, or gradually, as the result of an activity that persistently puts pressure on the perineum. Sudden damage to the perineum is called an acute injury, while gradual damage is called a chronic injury.

Why Is The Perineum Important?

The perineum is important because it contains blood vessels and nerves that supply the urinary tract and genitals with blood and nerve signals. The perineum lies just below a sheet of muscles called the pelvic floor muscles. Pelvic floor muscles support the bladder and bowel.

What Are The Complications Of Perineal Injury?

Injury to the blood vessels, nerves, and muscles in the perineum can lead to complications such as:

- bladder control problems
- sexual problems

Bladder control problems. The nerves in the perineum carry signals from the bladder to the spinal cord and brain, telling the brain when the bladder is full. Those same nerves carry signals from the brain to the bladder and pelvic floor muscles, directing those muscles to hold or release urine. Injury to those nerves can block or interfere with the signals, causing the bladder to squeeze at the wrong time or not to squeeze at all. Damage to the pelvic floor muscles can cause bladder and bowel control problems.

Sexual problems. The perineal nerves also carry signals between the genitals and the brain. Injury to those nerves can interfere with the sensations of sexual contact.

Signals from the brain direct the smooth muscles in the genitals to relax, causing greater blood flow into the penis. In men, damaged blood vessels can cause erectile dysfunction (ED), the inability to achieve or maintain an erection firm enough for sexual intercourse. An internal portion of the penis runs through the perineum and contains a section of the urethra. As a result, damage to the perineum may also injure the penis and urethra.

Common Causes Of Acute Perineal Injury

Straddle Injuries

Straddle injuries result from falls onto objects such as metal bars, pipes, or wooden rails, where the person's legs are on either side of the object and the perineum strikes the object forcefully. These injuries include motorcycle and bike riding accidents, saddle horn injuries during horseback riding, falls on playground equipment such as monkey bars, and gymnastic accidents on an apparatus such as the parallel bars or pommel horse.

In rare situations, a blunt injury to the perineum may burst a blood vessel inside the erectile tissue of the penis, causing a persistent partial erection that can last for days to years. This condition is called high-flow priapism. If not treated, ED may result.

Impalement

Impalement injuries may involve metal fence posts, rods, or weapons that pierce the perineum. Impalement is rare, although it may occur where moving equipment and pointed tools are in use, such as on farms or construction sites. Impalement can also occur as the result of a fall, such as from a tree or playground equipment, onto something sharp. Impalement injuries are most common in combat situations. If an impalement injury pierces the skin and muscles, the injured person needs immediate medical attention to minimize blood loss and repair the injury.

What Are The Most Common Causes Of Chronic Perineal Injury?

Chronic perineal injury most often results from a job-or sport-related practice—such as bike, motorcycle, or horseback riding—or a long-term condition such as chronic constipation.

Sitting on a narrow, saddle-style bike seat—which has a protruding "nose" in the front—places far more pressure on the perineum than sitting in a regular chair. In a regular chair, the flesh and bone of the buttocks partially absorb the pressure of sitting, and the pressure occurs farther toward the back than on a bike seat. The straddling position on a narrow seat pinches the perineal blood vessels and nerves, possibly causing blood vessel and nerve damage over time. Research shows wider, noseless seats reduce perineal pressure.

Occasional bike riding for short periods of time may pose no risk. However, men who ride bikes several hours a week—such as competitive bicyclists, bicycle couriers, and bicycle patrol officers—have a significantly higher risk of developing mild to severe ED. The ED may be caused by repetitive pressure on blood vessels, which constricts them and results in plaque buildup in the vessels.

Other activities that involve riding saddle-style include motorcycle and horseback riding. Researchers have studied bike riding more extensively than these other activities; however, the few studies published regarding motorcycle and horseback riding suggest motorcycle riding increases the risk of ED and urinary symptoms. Horseback riding appears relatively safe in terms of chronic injury, although the action of bouncing up and down, repeatedly striking the perineum, has the potential for causing damage.

How Is Perineal Injury Evaluated?

Healthcare providers evaluate perineal injury based on the circumstances and severity of the injury. In general, the evaluation process includes a physical examination and one or more imaging tests.

During a physical examination, the patient lies face-up with legs spread and feet in stirrups. The healthcare provider looks for cuts, bruises, or bleeding from the anus. The healthcare provider may insert a gloved, lubricated finger into the rectum to feel for internal injuries.

To look for internal injuries, the healthcare provider may order one or more imaging tests.

- Computerized tomography (CT)
- Magnetic resonance imaging (MRI)
- Ultrasound

How Is Perineal Injury Treated?

Treatments for perineal injury vary with the severity and type of injury. Tears or incisions may require stitches. Traumatic or piercing injuries may require surgery to repair damaged pelvic floor muscles, blood vessels, and nerves. Treatment for these acute injuries may also include antibiotics to prevent infection. After a healthcare provider stabilizes an acute injury so blood loss is no longer a concern, a person may still face some long-term effects of the injury, such as bladder control and sexual function problems. A healthcare provider can treat high-flow priapism caused by a blunt injury to the perineum with medication, blockage of the burst blood vessel under X-ray guidance, or surgery.

How Can Perineal Injury Be Prevented?

Preventing perineal injury requires being aware of and taking steps to minimize the dangers of activities such as construction work or bike riding:

- People should talk with their healthcare provider about the benefits and risks of perineal surgery well before the operation.

- People who play or work around moving equipment or sharp objects should wear protective gear whenever possible.

- People who ride bikes, motorcycles, or horses should find seats or saddles designed to place the most pressure on the buttocks and minimize pressure on the perineum. Many healthcare providers advise bike riders to use noseless bike seats and to ride in an upright position rather than lean over the handlebars. The National Institute for Occupational Safety and Health (NIOSH), part of the Centers for Disease Control and Prevention (CDC), recommends noseless seats for people who ride bikes as part of their job.

- People with constipation should talk with their healthcare provider about whether to take a laxative or stool softener to minimize straining during a bowel movement.

Using No-Nose (Noseless) Bicycle Saddles To Prevent Genital Numbness And Sexual Dysfunction

The National Institute for Occupational Safety and Health (NIOSH) conducted a study to examine the effect of bicycle saddle design on groin pressure. The study found that the traditional sport/racing saddle was associated with more than two times the pressure in the perineal region than the saddles without a protruding nose. There were no significant differences in perineal pressure among the no-nose saddles. Measures of weight distribution on the pedals and handlebars indicated no differences between the traditional saddle and those without protruding noses.

NIOSH recommends that workers who ride a bicycle as part of their job take the following steps to help prevent sexual and reproductive health problems:

- Use a no-nose saddle for workplace bicycling. Give yourself time to get used to riding with a no-nose saddle. At first, it may seem very different from the saddle you have used in the past. No-nose saddles may not always be available at retail bicycle shops, but they are readily available for purchase through the Internet.

- Seek guidance on proper bicycle fit from a trained bicycle fit specialist. Use of a no-nose saddle may require different saddle height and angle adjustments. Be sure that the no-nose saddle is adjusted according to the manufacturer's instructions.

- Dismount the bicycle when at a standstill. Do not lean against a post or other object to stay seated on the bicycle saddle when you are not riding.

- Dismount the bicycle if you begin to have numbness, tingling, or loss of feeling in any part of your body.

While much of the scientific community has reached a consensus about the association between erectile dysfunction and traditional bicycle saddles, no-nose saddle designs have not been universally embraced by many cyclists.

Chapter 49

Hip Injuries

What Is A Broken Hip?

A broken hip is a break in the thigh bone (called the "femur") near the hip joint. A broken hip can occur from falling or from daily use if the femur is weak. The femur is one of the strongest bones in your body, but it may weaken with age. Even a minor injury may cause the bone to break.

People who have a bone-weakening condition called "osteoporosis" are more likely to break a hip.

Many people are unaware of the link between a broken bone and osteoporosis. Osteoporosis, or "porous bone," is a disease characterized by low bone mass. It makes bones fragile and more prone to fractures, especially the bones of the hip, spine, and wrist. Osteoporosis is called a "silent disease" because bone loss occurs without symptoms. People typically do not know that they have osteoporosis until their bones become so weak that a sudden strain, twist, or fall results in a fracture.

(Source: "Once Is Enough: A Guide To Preventing Future Fractures," National Institute of Arthritis and Musculoskeletal and Skin Diseases (NIAMS).)

A broken hip is a serious injury that is very painful and can keep you from walking. People with broken hips may be at risk for other problems, such as pneumonia, blood clots, and

About This Chapter: Text under the heading "What Is A Broken Hip?" is excerpted from "Managing Pain From A Broken Hip: A Guide For Adults And Their Caregivers," Agency for Healthcare Research and Quality (AHRQ), U.S. Department of Health and Human Services (HHS), May 17, 2011. Reviewed July 2017; Text under the heading "Hip Fractures" is excerpted from "Treatment Of Common Hip Fractures," Agency for Healthcare Research and Quality (AHRQ), U.S. Department of Health and Human Services (HHS), August 2009. Reviewed July 2017.

muscle weakness. Some problems can be life threatening. For that reason, if possible, broken hips are treated with an operation to repair the hip, physical therapy to help you gain strength after the operation, and medicine to help ease the pain.

Hip Fractures

Hip fractures are generally classified into three major types, depending on the specific location of the fracture: femoral neck, intertrochanteric, and subtrochanteric fractures. The term pertrochanteric hip fracture may also be used in hip fracture literature and refers to a more inclusive set of extracapsular fractures, including intertrochanteric, subtrochanteric, and mixed fracture patterns.

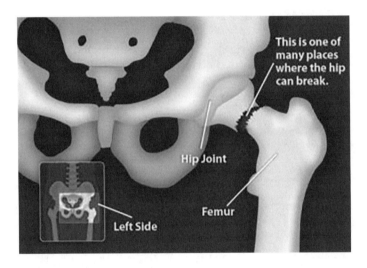

Figure 49.1. Hip Fracture

(Source: "Managing Pain From A Broken Hip: A Guide For Adults And Their Caregivers," Effective Health Care Program, Agency for Healthcare Research and Quality (AHRQ).)

Femoral neck fractures occur in the narrowed section of the upper femur between the rounded femoral head and bony projections called trochanters. Femoral neck fractures are grouped into *nondisplaced* and *displaced* fractures by the alignment of the fractured segments in relation to the original anatomic position of the femur.

Intertrochanteric hip fractures occur in the area between the greater and lesser trochanters. The trochanters are bony projections where major hip muscles attach. Intertrochanteric fractures may be further grouped into *stable* and *unstable* fractures, depending on the location, number, and size of the fractured bony segments.

Subtrochanteric fractures occur at or below the level of the lesser trochanter in the upper portion of the femur. Isolated subtrochanteric fractures occur in the area between the upper border of the lesser trochanter to 5 cm below it, toward the knee. Subtrochanteric fractures may include only a short, linear section of the proximal femur or maybe part of a larger fracture pattern that involves both the intertrochanteric and subtrochanteric sections of the femur. Orthopaedic surgeons differ on their definition of subtrochanteric fractures, and may also consider fractures that extend further toward the knee to be subtrochanteric.

The vast majority of hip fracture patients are treated with surgical repair. The short-term goal of surgical treatment is to stabilize the hip fracture enough to withstand early mobilization and weight bearing, which prevents complications due to prolonged bed rest and aids in fracture healing. The type of surgery is generally based on the fracture pattern and patient characteristics. Pertrochanteric fractures are generally managed with internal fixation, most often plate/screw devices or intramedullary nails. Femoral neck fractures are treated with either internal fixation or arthroplasty. Hemiarthroplasty replaces the femoral head segment of the upper femur with an artificial implant. The patient's own acetabulum is not replaced. Total hip arthroplasty is the prosthetic replacement of the entire hip joint, both the femoral head and the acetabulum within the pelvis.

The goal of treatment for hip fractures is to return patients to their prefracture level of function. There is a growing body of literature on treatment options and their effects on intermediary and patient postsurgical treatment outcomes, including several systematic reviews; however, no comprehensive organization of the evidence across all types of geriatric hip fractures exists.

Chapter 50

Knee Injuries

What Do The Knees Do?

The knees provide stable support for the body. They also allow the legs to bend and straighten. Both flexibility and stability are needed to stand, walk, run, crouch, jump, and turn. Other parts of the body help the knees do their job. These are:

- Bones
- Cartilage
- Muscles
- Ligaments
- Tendons

If any of these parts are injured, the knee may hurt and not be able to do its job.

Who Gets Knee Problems?

Men, women, and children can have knee problems. They occur in people of all races and ethnic backgrounds.

What Causes Knee Problems?

Mechanical knee problems can be caused by:

- A direct blow or sudden movements that strain the knee.

About This Chapter: This chapter includes text excerpted from "Fast Facts About Knee Problems," National Institute of Arthritis and Musculoskeletal and Skin Diseases (NIAMS), November 2014.

- Osteoarthritis in the knee, resulting from wear and tear on its parts.

Inflammatory knee problems can be caused by certain rheumatic diseases, such as rheumatoid arthritis and systemic lupus erythematosus (lupus). These diseases cause swelling that can damage the knees permanently.

How Are Knee Problems Diagnosed?

Doctors diagnose knee problems by using:

- Medical history

- Physical examination

- Diagnostic tests (such as X-rays, bone scan, computed tomography scan [CAT scan], magnetic resonance imaging [MRI], arthroscopy, and biopsy)

Types Of Knee Problems

Arthritis In The Knees

The most common type of arthritis of the knee is osteoarthritis. In this disease, the cartilage in the knee gradually wears away. Treatments for osteoarthritis are:

- Medicines to reduce pain, such as aspirin and acetaminophen

- Medicines to reduce swelling and inflammation, such as ibuprofen and nonsteroidal anti-inflammatory drugs (NSAIDs)

- Exercises to improve movement and strength

- Weight loss

Rheumatoid arthritis is another type of arthritis that affects the knee. In rheumatoid arthritis, the knee becomes inflamed and cartilage may be destroyed. Treatment includes:

- Physical therapy

- Medications

- Knee replacement surgery (for a seriously damaged knee)

Cartilage Injuries And Disorders

Chondromalacia occurs when the cartilage of the knee cap softens. This can be caused by injury, overuse, or muscle weakness, or if parts of the knee are out of alignment. Chondromalacia can develop if a blow to the knee cap tears off a piece of cartilage or a piece of cartilage containing a bone fragment.

The meniscus is a C-shaped piece of cartilage that acts like a pad between the femur (thigh bone) and tibia (shin bone). It is easily injured if the knee is twisted while bearing weight. A partial or total tear may occur. If the tear is tiny, the meniscus stays connected to the front and back of the knee. If the tear is large, the meniscus may be left hanging by a thread of cartilage. The seriousness of the injury depends on the location and the size of the tear.

Treatment for cartilage injuries includes:

- Exercises to strengthen muscles

- Electrical stimulation to strengthen muscles

- Surgery for severe injuries

Ligament Injuries

Two commonly injured ligaments in the knee are the anterior cruciate ligament (ACL) and the posterior cruciate ligament (PCL). An injury to these ligaments is sometimes called a "sprain." The ACL is most often stretched or torn (or both) by a sudden twisting motion. The PCL is usually injured by a direct impact, such as in an automobile accident or football tackle.

The medial and lateral collateral ligaments are usually injured by a blow to the outer side of the knee. This can stretch and tear a ligament. These blows frequently occur in sports such as football or hockey.

Ligament injuries are treated with:

- Ice packs (right after the injury) to reduce swelling

- Exercises to strengthen muscles

- A brace

- Surgery (for more severe injuries)

Tendon Injuries And Disorders

The three main types of tendon injuries and disorders are:

- Tendinitis and ruptured tendons

- Osgood-Schlatter disease

- Iliotibial band syndrome

Tendon injuries range from tendinitis (inflammation of a tendon) to a ruptured (torn) tendon. Torn tendons most often occur from:

- Overusing a tendon (particularly in some sports). The tendon stretches like a worn-out rubber band and becomes inflamed.

- Trying to break a fall. If thigh muscles contract, the tendon can tear. This is most likely to happen in older people with weak tendons.

One type of tendinitis of the knee is called jumper's knee. In sports that require jumping, such as basketball, the tendon can become inflamed or can tear.

Osgood-Schlatter disease is caused by stress or tension on part of the growth area of the upper shin bone. It causes swelling in the knee and upper part of the shin bone. It can happen if a person's tendon tears away from the bone, taking a piece of bone with it. Young people who run and jump while playing sports can have this type of injury.

Iliotibial band syndrome occurs when a tendon rubs over the outer bone of the knee causing swelling. It happens if the knee is overused for a long time. This sometimes occurs in sports training.

Treatment for tendon injuries and disorders includes:

- Rest

- Ice

- Elevation

- Medicines such as aspirin or ibuprofen to relieve pain and reduce swelling

- Limiting sports activity

- Exercise for stretching and strengthening

- A cast, if there is a partial tear

- Surgery for complete tears or very severe injuries

Other Knee Injuries

Osteochondritis dissecans occurs when not enough blood goes to part of the bone under a joint surface. The bone and cartilage gradually loosen and cause pain. Some cartilage may break off and cause sharp pain, weakness, and locking of the joint. A person with this condition may develop osteoarthritis. Surgery is the main treatment.

- If cartilage fragments have not broken loose, a surgeon may pin or screw them in place. This can stimulate new blood flow to the cartilage.

- If fragments are loose, the surgeon may scrape the cavity to reach fresh bone and add a bone graft to fix the fragments in position.

- Research is being done to investigate cartilage and tissue transplants.

Plica syndrome occurs when bands of tissue in the knee called plicae swell from overuse or injury. Treatments for this syndrome are:

- Medicines such as aspirin or ibuprofen to reduce swelling

- Rest

- Ice

- Elastic bandage on the knee

- Exercises to strengthen muscles

- Cortisone injection into the plicae

- Surgery to remove the plicae if the first treatments do not fix the problem.

What Kinds Of Doctors Treat Knee Problems?

Injuries and diseases of the knees are usually treated by an orthopaedist (a doctor who treats problems with bones, joints, ligaments, tendons, and muscles).

How Can People Prevent Knee Problems?

Some knee problems (such as those resulting from an accident) can't be prevented. But many knee problems can be prevented by doing the following:

- Warm up before playing sports. Walking and stretching are good warm-up exercises. Stretching the muscles in the front and the back of the thighs is a good way to warm up the knees.

- Make the leg muscles strong by doing certain exercises (for example, walking up stairs, riding a stationary bicycle, or working out with weights).

- Avoid sudden changes in the intensity of exercise.

- Increase the force or duration of activity slowly.

- Wear shoes that fit and are in good condition.

- Maintain a healthy weight. Extra weight puts pressure on the knees.

Avoiding Knee Injuries

Knee injuries happen pretty often to young people. One of the most common knee injuries is a torn anterior cruciate ligament, called ACL for short. Teenage girls get these injuries a lot more than guys do. Why? Possibly because of the way girls' bodies are made or because of the way girls use them.

If you have a torn ACL, you might have one or all of the following symptoms:

- A "popping" sound at the time of the injury
- Pain
- Not being able to put weight on your knee
- Swelling

If you think you have any kind of injury to your knee, you should stop using it. Tell your parent or guardian right away (or, if you are at school, tell your coach or teacher). Treatment for a torn ACL may include surgery and physical therapy. Don't play again until your doctor says you can.

Your best bet is to try to prevent an ACL injury. Talk to your coach or gym teacher about what you can do. Special exercises can help build strength and flexibility, for example. You also can learn safer ways to do riskier movements, like making sure to bend your knees when you jump.

(Source: "Avoiding Injuries," girlshealth.gov, Office on Women's Health (OWH).)

What Types Of Exercise Are Best For Someone With Knee Problems?

Three types of exercise are best for people with arthritis in the knees:

1. Range-of-motion exercises. These exercises help maintain or increase flexibility. They also help relieve stiffness in the knee.

2. Strengthening exercises. These exercises help maintain or increase muscle strength. Strong muscles help support and protect joints with arthritis.

3. Aerobic or endurance exercises. These exercises improve heart function and blood circulation. They also help control weight. Some studies show that aerobic exercise can reduce swelling in some joints.

Chapter 51

Shin Splints

Medial tibial stress syndrome, commonly called shin splints, is characterized by inflammation of the muscles, tendons, and bone tissue around the tibia, the larger of the two bones in the lower leg below the knee. Although most common among runners, shin splints can be caused by any vigorous sports activity or a sudden increase in the intensity of your training routine. Shin splints may also be caused by hyperpronation of the foot. Commonly called "flat feet," hyperpronation causes an individual's weight to shift from the heel to the forefeet. This in turn, places a stress on the muscles, tendons, and ligaments of the foot, shin, and knee and precipitates overuse injuries in high impact sports such as running, basketball, and soccer.

Risk Factors Of Shin Splints

Runners, gymnasts, and military recruits are most commonly affected by shin splints, but even walkers can develop shin splints, especially if they walk too much, or too fast. Athletes who start a new program and those who rapidly increase the duration and intensity of activity are also at risk for developing shin splints. Certain preexisting conditions such as weak core muscles and muscle imbalance can also trigger shin splints as can flat feet and high foot arches. Training on hard, uneven surfaces, such as concrete or wearing improper, worn out shoes that do not provide arch support can also cause shin splints or exacerbate the condition.

Symptoms Of Shin Splints

Tenderness and pain along the shin bone in one or both legs caused by inflammation of the periosteum (the connective tissue sheath around the tibia) and the soft tissues surrounding it

"Shin Splints," © 2017 Omnigraphics. Reviewed July 2017.

are typical of a shin splint. What begins as a dull, diffuse ache in the lower leg during exercise and improves considerably with cessation of activity may progress to sharp, severe pain which persists even during inactivity. In extreme cases, untreated shin splints can lead to stress fractures of the tibia. This may show up as acute, focal pain that makes it difficult to continue any activity.

Diagnosis Of Shin Splints

A shin splint is usually diagnosed on the basis of a physical examination and medical history. However, the doctor may order imaging tests to eliminate other possible causes including peripheral vascular disease, exertional compartment syndrome, or tendinitis. If the doctor suspects the shin splint has progressed to a stress fracture, he may order magnetic resonance imaging (MRI) to evaluate the extent of tibial injury and any associated soft tissue injury.

Treatment For Shin Splints

Conservative treatment options for shin splints include rest and ice. Rest is regarded as the most important treatment during the acute phase of injury and depending on the severity of condition, patients may be advised cessation of activity for 2–6 weeks. NSAIDs (nonsteroidal anti-inflammatory drugs) and Acetaminophen are prescribed for pain relief. Applying an ice pack for 15–20 minutes at a time is advised several times a day. An elastic compression bandage around the shin may also be useful in bringing down the swelling.

The second phase of treatment focuses on modifying training routines and correcting biomechanical abnormalities such as flat foot. Physical therapists and podiatrists can also work with athletes to formulate an appropriate rehabilitation plan to enable their return to sports. The plan can involve low-impact exercises; gait retraining; proper technique; and correct warm-up routines. Return to activity at a lower level intensity is the most important aspect of a proper rehabilitation plan. Calf exercises to strengthen the calf muscles and prevent muscle fatigue improve endurance. Cross-training exercises such as swimming and cycling can also be added to the rehab regimen. At the same time care should be taken to scale back any activity that exacerbates the condition.

Athletic Footwear And Orthotics

Appropriate footwear may be required to reduce load on the shin, and some athletes, especially those with excessive pronation or fallen arches, may benefit from custom-made orthotics which can help stabilize the foot and ankle.

Surgery

The majority of shin splint cases are cured or improve significantly with conservative treatment, and surgery is considered only in cases that do not benefit from conservative management. Fasciotomy, in which an incision is made in the fascia—the tissue covering the calf muscle sheath—can be helpful when the shin splint is caused by a damaged fascia. Surgery may also be used to treat shin splints caused by the inflammation of the periosteum, and the procedure involves stripping of the periosteum.

If the shin splint has progressed to a high risk stress fracture, surgery with intramedullary nail placement (a metal rod placed in the cavity of a bone) is considered. Returning to sports after surgery usually takes many months. The surgeon has to determine, with the help of imaging tests, if the fracture has healed before he or she can allow the athlete to bear weight. An extensive rehabilitation program to rebuild strength and regain full weight bearing precedes the athlete's gradual return to sports.

References

1. "Shin Splints," American Academy of Orthopaedic Surgeons (AAOS), 2012.

2. "Shin Splints," Mayo Clinic, 2016.

3. "Medial Tibial Stress Syndrome: Conservative Treatment Options," National Institute of Health (NIH), 2009.

Chapter 52

Foot Injuries

Metatarsalgia

The metatarsals are five long bones that form the arch in the middle of the foot. They connect to the toe bones at the ball of the foot. Metatarsalgia is a condition in which the heads of the metatarsal bones near the toe joints rub together, putting pressure on nerves and causing pain and inflammation in the ball of the foot. It is sometimes referred to as a stone bruise because the stabbing pain may resemble having a rock in the shoe. Metatarsalgia often develops as an overuse injury in athletes who participate in sports that involve running and jumping, although it can also affect people who have underlying foot issues or wear improperly fitting shoes.

Causes And Risk Factors Of Metatarsalgia

Several different activity and lifestyle factors appear to be related to the development of metatarsalgia. In addition, certain physical traits and medical conditions appear to increase people's risk. Some of the most common causes and risk factors include the following:

- participating in high-impact sports, such as distance running or dance;
- wearing shoes that fit poorly, lack support and cushioning, or place pressure on the ball of the foot, such as high heels, pointy or box-toe shoes, and cleats or spikes;
- having feet with high arches or a second toe that is longer than the big toe;
- having deformities of the feet, such as hammertoes or bunions;

- being overweight;

- reaching middle age, when the pad of fat that protects the ball of the foot naturally becomes thinner and provides less protection from impact;

- developing stress fractures in the metatarsals, which can lead to metatarsalgia when people adjust the weight distribution in their feet to compensate;

- having inflammatory conditions such as gout or rheumatoid arthritis;

- having diabetes, which can irritate nerves in the feet;

- developing Morton's neuroma, a condition in which fibrous tissue grows between the metatarsal heads.

Symptoms And Diagnosis Of Metatarsalgia

The main symptom of metatarsalgia is pain in the ball of the foot. The pain may be described as sharp, shooting, aching, burning, or like having a rock in the shoe. It typically becomes worse upon standing, walking, running, jumping, or flexing the feet. Walking barefoot on a hard surface may be particularly painful. Some people also experience numbness or tingling in the toes. The symptoms typically appear gradually and get worse over time, until the pain makes it difficult for athletes to compete to their level of ability.

To diagnose metatarsalgia, the doctor will begin by asking questions about the patient's symptoms, lifestyle and activities, and usual footwear. The doctor may also watch the patient walk on a treadmill to assess their normal gait and determine whether the placement of the feet is putting excess pressure on the metatarsal heads. The doctor may order blood tests to see whether the patient has an underlying medical condition that increases the risk of metatarsalgia, such as gout, diabetes, or arthritis. Finally, the doctor is likely to order diagnostic imaging tests such as X-rays or a magnetic resonance imaging (MRI) scan to check for stress fractures or structural problems in the foot.

Treatment Of Metatarsalgia

Most cases of metatarsalgia respond to conservative methods of treatment, such as the following:

- taking a break from high-impact sports and other activities that cause pain, and switch to low-impact cross-training options like swimming or bicycling to maintain fitness;

- applying ice to the affected foot several times per day;

- elevating the foot whenever possible to reduce swelling;

- taking anti-inflammatory medications to relieve pain and swelling;

- avoiding wearing high heels or shoes that do not fit properly;

- replacing running shoes regularly;

- using metatarsal pads, shock-absorbing insoles, or arch supports to relieve pressure on the metatarsal bones and improve foot function.

For severe cases of metatarsalgia that do not improve with conservative treatment, a doctor may try a steroid injection to help alleviate pain and inflammation. Surgery is considered a treatment of last resort for the condition. Procedures used to treat metatarsalgia may involve reshaping the metatarsal bones, releasing or removing irritated nerves between the metatarsal bones, or correcting other foot deformities that may be contributing to the condition, such as hammertoes or bunions. Left untreated, metatarsalgia can cause alterations in foot placement or gait that can lead to future problems with the ankles, knees, hips, or back.

Sesamoiditis And Sesamoid Fracture

A sesamoid is a special type of bone that is embedded within a muscle or tendon rather than connected to another bone at a joint. Sesamoid bones appear in several parts of the human body, including the hand, wrist, knee, and foot. There are two sesamoid bones located on the underside of the ball of the foot—one on each side of the first metatarsal bone where it meets the big toe. They are embedded in the flexor hallucis brevis tendon, which helps control the up-and-down motion of the big toe. As the tendon slides over the smooth surface of the sesamoid bones, it acts like a pulley to enable the big toe to push off the ground and absorb impact from the ground while walking or running.

The sesamoid bones in the foot are vulnerable to several types of injury:

- Sesamoiditis is an overuse injury that is common among athletes who engage in sports and activities that put constant pressure or repeated force on the forefoot, such as running, dancing, or squatting in the catcher position in baseball. The rubbing of the tendon on the sesamoid bones causes irritation and chronic inflammation.

- Sesamoid fracture is when one or both of the sesamoid bones in the foot are broken. An acute sesamoid fracture may occur due to a traumatic injury, such as falling from a height and landing on the ball of the foot, while a chronic sesamoid fracture may occur due to repetitive stress.

Turf toe is a soft tissue injury of the big toe that sometimes affects the sesamoid bones or the flexor hallucis brevis tendon. It typically occurs due to traumatic hyperextension of the big toe, and it often affects athletes who play sports on grass, like football or soccer.

Symptoms And Diagnosis Of Sesamoiditis And Sesamoid Fracture

The main symptom of sesamoid injury is pain in the ball of the foot at the base of the big toe. In sesamoiditis, the pain is likely to appear gradually over time and become worse with activity. In a sesamoid fracture, the pain is more likely to appear suddenly and be accompanied by swelling, bruising, and limited range of motion of the big toe. In turf toe, the pain and swelling may tend to affect the toe itself more than the ball of the foot.

To diagnose a sesamoid injury, the doctor will examine the foot for signs of inflammation and tenderness and assess the range of motion in the big toe. An X-ray is usually performed to check for a sesamoid fracture. In some cases, however, X-rays may not aid in diagnosis because the patient has bipartite sesamoid bones, meaning that the bones are naturally divided into two pieces. Since the sesamoid bones are so small, it can be difficult to distinguish between bipartite sesamoid bones and a sesamoid fracture. The radiologist is likely to concentrate on the edges of the bones, which tend to be smooth in a bipartite sesamoid and jagged in a fractured sesamoid. An X-ray of the other foot can also be used for comparison. Finally, the doctor may order blood tests to check for underlying medical conditions that can cause pain and inflammation in the feet, such as arthritis or gout.

Treatment Of Sesamoiditis And Sesamoid Fracture

Sesamoiditis usually improves after several weeks of conservative, noninvasive treatment. Athletes are typically advised to take a break from physical activities that cause pain, apply ice to the bottom of the foot, and use anti-inflammatory medication to relieve pain and swelling. It may also be helpful to wear low-heeled shoes with stiff soles and to insert a cushioning pad made of felt or foam rubber to reduce pressure on the ball of the foot and big toe. The toe may also be immobilized with athletic tape in a downward-bending or flexed position to promote healing.

Treatment for sesamoid fracture usually involves immobilization of the foot in a walking cast or removable fracture brace for six to eight weeks. To reduce swelling, the doctor may inject a steroid medication into the metatarsophalangeal joint at the base of the big toe.

If this conservative treatment fails to relieve pain and restore function to the foot, surgery may be necessary. The most common procedure used to treat a sesamoid fracture is sesamoidectomy, or surgical removal of the broken sesamoid bones. Surgery is considered a last resort, however, due to the risk of complications—such as damage to the soft tissues or joint capsule of the metatarsophalangeal joint—that can affect foot function. Removal of the sesamoid bones can also result in misalignment of the foot and the development of an uncomfortable foot deformity called a bunion. These large, bony lumps on the side of the foot occur when weakness in the joint causes the big toe to twist toward the middle of the foot.

Fifth Metatarsal Fracture

The metatarsals are a group of five long bones located in the forefoot. They connect the articulating bones of the mid- and hind-foot to the phalanges (toe bones) and constitute an important weight-bearing structure. The five metatarsals are numbered from the big toe as the first, second, third, fourth and fifth metatarsal, each consisting of a body or shaft, a proximal base, and a distal head. Fractures of the metatarsal are quite common, often resulting from trauma or direct injury, such as dropping a heavy object on the foot or kicking something hard. Fractures can also result from chronic overuse or repetitive stress injury, commonly associated with high-impact sports, such as soccer, football, or running.

The fifth metatarsal, the bone that connects to the little toe, is the most commonly fractured metatarsal. Injury can occur at any point along the length of the bone and usually results from inversion (movement that tilts the foot toward the midline of the body) or dorsiflexion (backward bending of the foot). Depending on the extent and mechanism of the injury, metatarsal fractures may be closed or open. In a closed fracture, the overlying skin is intact, and there is no open wound. An open fracture, on the other hand, is accompanied by damage to skin and soft tissue and is usually associated with risk of infection. Fractures of the fifth metatarsal can also be categorized as displaced or nondisplaced. In a nondisplaced fracture, the bone maintains its alignment despite being broken into fragments. In contrast, a displaced fracture results in an incorrect alignment of the bone fragments making it more difficult to treat.

Types Of Metatarsal Fracture

Three types of fractures can occur in the fifth metatarsal:

- **Avulsion fracture.** This type of fracture usually occurs at the base of the fifth metatarsal. A violent force may cause the tendon or ligament that attaches to the base of the metatarsal to pull away a fragment from the main bone. Also called the "dancer's fracture," avulsion fractures may co-occur with ankle sprains, and ankle fractures and may need to be evaluated alongside ankle injuries to avoid a missed diagnosis. Symptoms can include ecchymosis (discoloration of skin from hemorrhage underneath), soft tissue swelling, and pain at the base of the metatarsal. Nondisplaced avulsion fractures are generally treated conservatively, and the prognosis is usually good. Displaced avulsion fractures, by and large, require surgical intervention.

- **Jones fracture.** Named after the English surgeon and Father of Modern Orthopedics, Sir Robert Jones, a Jones fracture is the most complex of the fifth metatarsal fractures and occurs within 1.5 cm of the tuberosity (a rounded bump at the end of the bone). This type of injury is ascribed to an acute trauma caused by sudden pivot-shifting with the heel off the ground and is commonly experienced in sports such as basketball, football, and tennis. Typical symptoms of Jones Fracture include the sudden onset of pain, swelling, and weight-bearing difficulty. In addition to difficulty walking, there is pain associated with other types of increased activity. One of the most significant factors that affects the treatment outcome for Jones fracture is the poor blood supply to the injured area. Some parts of the fifth metatarsal have poor vascularity and therefore a propensity for delayed healing.

- **Stress fracture.** Stress fractures are the least common type of the fifth metatarsal fractures and are precipitated by fatigue or repetitive stress, especially in young athletes. These fractures are often the result of poor conditioning, but improper technique and equipment are also risk factors for this type of injury. In those starting out a new exercise regimen, doing too much too soon can raise the risk of stress fractures significantly. Experienced athletes are also at risk when they tend to overdo training or play without giving their body a chance to recover. Although the exact mechanism of stress fractures of the fifth metatarsal remains unclear, it is believed that prolonged muscle fatigue transmits excessive forces to the surrounding bone, thereby reducing its stress-bearing capacity. Stress fractures can result in significant morbidity for athletes if diagnosis and treatment are delayed. The symptoms usually present as pain for weeks or months, with the intensity of pain increasing with weight-bearing activity.

Diagnosis Of Metatarsal Fracture

As with any type of fracture, physical examination and patient history are the first steps in diagnosis. Physical examination focuses on external signs of injury; palpation for assessing the point of greatest pain, and neurovascular evaluation. Patient history would typically include the cause of the injury, as well as the onset and duration of symptoms.

Imaging Tests

Radiography is the mainstay of diagnosis of fifth metatarsal injuries. While most fractures show up on X-rays, some of them may require CT (computed tomography) or MRI (magnetic resonance imaging) scans for further assessment. Metatarsal stress fractures are generally more difficult to investigate than other types of fractures, as they often don't show up on X-rays, particularly in the early stages. Consequently, a bone scan or MRI may be needed to make a stress-fracture diagnosis.

Treatment Of Metatarsal Fracture

The symptoms, location, and extent of injury will determine the type of treatment for fractures of the fifth metatarsal. Typically, nonsurgical intervention is considered for nondisplaced fractures, including weight-bearing protection in a cast or CAM (controlled ankle movement) boot. Crutches may also be used to take the weight off the injured foot. Pain usually subsides within eight weeks following injury. Surgical intervention is considered for displaced fractures or those that fail to heal following conservative treatment. Surgery is generally the preferred treatment option for Jones and stress fractures in athletes who are looking for a quick return-to-play without much weight-bearing restriction. The gold standard in surgical treatment involves fixation of an intramedullary screw. With this procedure, a small incision is made on the outer side of the foot, and the fractured pieces of the bones are aligned. A hole is then drilled through the metatarsal shaft, and a surgical screw is inserted through the two ends of the fractured bone to stabilize the fracture. In some cases, the procedure may be accompanied by bone grafting to hasten bone union and reduce the risk of refracture.

References

1. "Fractures of the Fifth Metatarsal," American College of Foot and Ankle Surgeons (ACFAS), n.d.

2. Johnson, Julie, MD. "Fifth Metatarsal Fractures," American Orthopaedic Foot and Ankle Society (AOFAS), June 2015.

3. Strayer, Scott M., MC, Steven G. Greece, MD, and Michael J. Petrizzi, MD. "Fractures of the Proximal Fifth Metatarsal," American Academy of Family Physicians (AAFP), May 1, 1999.

4. Bowes, Julia, MD and Richard Buckley, MD. "Fifth Metatarsal Fractures and Current Treatment," National Center for Biotechnology Information (NCBI), December 18, 2016.

5. "Metatarsalgia," Mayo Clinic, November 4, 2016.

6. "Metatarsalgia," WebMD, 2017.

7. Nordqvist, Christian. "Metatarsalgia: Causes, Symptoms, and Treatments," *Medical News Today*, June 18, 2015.

8. "Sesamoid Injuries," American Orthopaedic Foot and Ankle Society (AOFAS), 2017.

9. "Sesamoid Injuries in the Foot," Foot Health Facts, 2017.

10. Swierzewski, John J. "Sesamoiditis," Remedy's Health Communities, December 31, 1999.

Chapter 53

Ankle Injuries

Ankle Sprains

Your ankle bone and the ends of your two lower leg bones make up the ankle joint. Your ligaments, which connect bones to one another, stabilize and support it. Your muscles and tendons move it. The most common ankle problems are sprains and fractures. A sprain is an injury to the ligaments. It may take a few weeks to many months to heal completely.

Risk Factors

Ankle sprains are the most common acute pathology seen in athletic activities. Up to one-sixth of all time lost from sports is because of this type of injury. Sixteen percent of all sports injuries are ankle ligament sprains. The cost for treatment and rehabilitation of these injuries is significant. Reducing the incidence of ankle ligament injuries depends on identifying the conditions under which such injuries occur (e.g., extrinsic variables, such as height and ankle-specific measures, that might predispose athletes to such injuries). Many researchers have reported that individuals with a history of ankle sprains are more susceptible to subsequent ankle sprains or chronic ankle instability. Studies show that over 70 percent of ankle sprains occur in ankles that had previously been sprained. Therefore, previously sprained ankles must have some risk factors that cause them to be recurrently sprained. Numerous factors and mechanisms are thought to contribute to this increased ankle sprain occurrence. Some of these

About This Chapter: Text in this chapter begins with excerpts from "Ankle Injuries And Disorders," National Institutes of Health (NIH), March 17, 2016; Text under the heading "Risk Factors" is excerpted from "Balance Problems After Unilateral Lateral Ankle Sprains," U.S. Department of Veterans Affairs (VA), December 2006. Reviewed July 2017; Text beginning with the heading "Symptoms" is excerpted from "Protocols For Injuries To The Foot And Ankle," Rhode Island Judiciary, U.S. Department of Justice (DOJ), May 5, 2009. Reviewed July 2017.

factors are instability, muscle weakness, limited mobility of the ankle joint, problems related to footwear, and damage to the proprioceptors in the ligaments of the ankle.

Symptoms

The patient typically presents acutely after an accident or fall with immediate pain and swelling at the injury site, with often the inability to ambulate. Obtaining an accurate history is important, in particular the mechanism of injury. Ankle sprains typically occur after an inversion of the foot ("rolling in," "rolled over"). The patient complains of pain and inability to ambulate.

Diagnosis

Radiography: Three view X-rays (AP, Mortise, and Lateral) should be obtained of the ankle to evaluate for injury. Stress views and weight bearing views can often be helpful to evaluate for gross ligamentous instability. Repeat X-rays 2–3 weeks after injury can be helpful in identifying stress fractures or unstable ligamentous injuries in those patients who fail to improve after a period of activity modification.

Treatment Based On Injury Type

Anatomy Of The Ankle

Stability of the ankle is made possible by both bony congruence (the fit of the talus within the distal tibia and fibula) as well as by the integrity of the ligaments, muscles, and tendons which surround the ankle. The ligaments and bones represent the static stabilizers (as they are fixed) and the muscles and tendons represent the dynamic stabilizers (as they move). The lateral side of the ankle is stabilized by the lateral collateral ligament (LCL) complex, the fibula and syndesmosis, and the peroneal tendons. The LCL complex consists of the anterior talo-fibular ligament, the calcaneo-fibular ligament, and the posterior talo-fibular ligament. The medial side of the ankle is stabilized by the deltoid ligament, the medial malleolus, the posterior tibial tendon, flexor digitorum longus tendon, and the flexor hallucis longus tendon. The deltoid ligament consists of superfi cial and deep layers which work in concert to stabilize the medial side of the ankle.

Grading Of Ankle Sprains

The most common ligament injured in the typical inversion ankle sprain is the anterior talo-fibular ligament, followed by the calcaneo-fibular ligament, the posterior talo-fibular ligament, and finally the deltoid ligament.

Ankle sprains are graded 1–3.

Acute surgical repair is NOT indicated, even with MRI confirmed complete ligament rupture. Patients with clinical ankle instability after months of rehabilitation MAY warrant surgical reconstruction.

1. **Grade 1 Sprain:** Microtearing of the collateral ligaments about the ankle, without any appreciable ankle joint laxity on exam. Treated with RICE protocol (Rest, Ice, Compressive Dressing (splint), Elevation). Typically resolves within 1–2 weeks.

2. **Grade 2 Sprain:** Complete tearing of some of the collateral ligaments of the ankle, with some laxity noted on physical exam. Treated with RICE protocol, immobilization with an ankle brace or CAM walker boot, and early mobilization with Physical Therapy. Typically resolved in 2–4 weeks.

3. **Grade 3 Sprain:** Complete rupture of the collateral ligaments of the ankle (usually medial or lateral side), with gross instability on examination. Acute surgical repair is NOT indicated. Treatment requires immobilization in a short leg cast or CAM walker boot for 2–3 weeks, followed by 3–6 weeks of Physical Therapy. Grade 3 sprains can potentially go on to gross instability that requires long-term bracing, rehabilitation, or surgical reconstruction.

Chronic Ankle Instability

Ankles which are chronically unstable after 2–3 months of rehabilitation and bracing warrant further workup with stress X-rays and/or MRI to evaluate for intra-articular osteochondral defects. Based on functional complaints, physical exam, and diagnostic tests, reconstructive surgery may be required for functional recovery. Postoperatively, patients are typically immobilized with a cast or CAM walker for 4–6 weeks, followed by a functional rehabilitation and Proprioceptive training program for another 4–6 weeks.

Return To Activity

For all of the above, return to sedentary work is possible as early as 1–2 weeks after injury or reconstructive surgery. Return to full function is based on completion of a functional rehabilitation and Proprioceptive training program.

Chapter 54

Plantar Fasciitis (Heel Spurs)

The plantar facia is a ligament that runs along the bottom of the foot, from the heel to the base of the toes. It provides support to the arch and helps absorb shock from walking, running, or jumping. Plantar fasciitis is a condition in which the plantar fascia becomes irritated and inflamed, causing pain in the heel. It is very common, affecting about 10 percent of all people at some point in their lives. Although it occurs most frequently among middle-aged people—especially women—it can also be related to overuse or repetitive stress among younger people who are active in sports.

Causes

Plantar fasciitis occurs when the ligament is subjected to strain or injury. The following situations increase the risk of developing the condition:

- having orthopedic issues like high arches or flat feet

- wearing shoes that are worn out, fit poorly, or have insufficient cushioning or arch support

- standing, walking, or running on hard surfaces for long periods of time

- rapidly increasing the intensity, distance, or duration of physical activity

- being overweight or experiencing sudden weight gain, such as during pregnancy

- using poor biomechanics or having an abnormal walking or running gait

- having tight Achilles tendons or calf muscles.

"Plantar Fasciitis (Heel Spurs)," © 2017 Omnigraphics. Reviewed July 2017.

Symptoms And Diagnosis

Pain on the bottom of the foot, usually on or just in front of the heel, is the most common symptom of plantar fasciitis. Many people find that the pain is most intense first thing in the morning, when they get out of bed and try to walk. Although the pain generally gets better during the day, it may grow worse again following physical activity. Stiffness in the foot may make it difficult to climb stairs or stand on tiptoes. The condition may affect only one foot or both feet at the same time.

To diagnose plantar fasciitis, the doctor will take a medical history, including questions about the symptoms the patient is experiencing, any injuries to the foot or heel, and the physical activities the patient engages in regularly. The doctor will also conduct a physical examination of the feet, checking for redness, swelling, and tenderness in the plantar fascia when flexing the foot or pointing the toe. In some cases, the doctor will also order diagnostic imaging tests, such as an X-ray or magnetic resonance imaging (MRI) scan, to rule out other types of foot injuries that could cause similar symptoms, such as a fracture.

Treatment

Many people see improvement in the symptoms of plantar fasciitis by using some combination of the following conservative approaches to treatment:

- Avoid activities that cause pain—such as standing or running on hard surfaces—for several weeks;

- Reduce inflammation by applying ice to the heel regularly and taking anti-inflammatory medications;

- Gently stretch the feet and Achilles tendons several times per day, beginning first thing in the morning before getting out of bed;

- Wear well-fitting shoes with cushioned soles and good arch support.

If conservative treatment approaches do not relieve symptoms, there are a few medical treatments available for plantar fasciitis. However, most of these treatments are relatively unproven, so they are mainly tried in difficult cases. For instance, a podiatrist can provide orthotic shoe inserts or heel cups to support the arches or correct other foot problems that may be contributing to the condiion. The doctor may also provide a splint to be worn overnight that holds the Achilles tendon and plantar fascia in a slightly stretched position. In some cases, the patient may be fitted with a walking brace or cast to cushion, protect, and rest the plantar fascia.

For patients with severe heel pain that continues for more than six months despite conservative treatments, the doctor may try an experimental approach called extracorporeal shock-wave therapy, which involves using an ultrasound device to deliver high-energy sound waves to the plantar fascia to promote healing. A steroid injection may also help relieve heel pain, although this treatment approach carries the risk of rupturing the plantar fascia. Surgery is considered the treatment of last resort for plantar fasciitis. The procedure involves partially detaching or releasing the plantar fascia from the heel bone and removing any bony growths known as heel spurs that may be present. Potential complications include weakness in the arch of the foot, damage to nerves in the foot, and loss of foot function.

Recovery And Prevention

Fortunately, most people recover from plantar fasciitis with rest and conservative treatment, although it may take several months for the symptoms to resolve. Physical therapy can speed the recovery process by stretching and strengthening muscles in the feet and lower legs, as well as correcting foot and gait problems that may have contributed to the condition.

Left untreated, however, plantar fasciitis can lead to chronic heel pain and a related condition called heel spurs. As the plantar fascia ligament is overstretched and irritated, the heel bone may respond by building up calcium deposits at the point where it attaches. Over time, these bony protrusions can erode the fatty tissue lining the bottom of the heel. Heel spurs can cause stabbing pain, damage to the foot, and gait changes that may in turn cause injury to the ankles, knees, hips, or back. It is important to note that plantar fasciitis is not typically caused by heel spurs, though, and that heel spurs are painless for most people.

The following steps can help prevent the development of plantar fasciitis:

- Wear shoes with cushioned heels and good arch support;
- Replace running shoes regularly;
- Warm up properly and stretch the Achilles tendon before exercise;
- Avoid prolonged standing, walking, or running on hard surfaces;
- Lose weight if needed.

References

1. Case-Lo, Christine. "Plantar Fasciitis," Healthline, February 16, 2016.

2. Imm, Nick. "Heel And Foot Pain (Plantar Fasciitis)," Patient, February 2, 2016.

3. "Plantar Fasciitis: Topic Overview," WebMD, 2015.

Part Four
Caring For Injured Athletes

Chapter 55

What To Do If A Sports Injury Occurs

Significant health benefits are derived from sports and recreational physical activities. Many people, from young children to adults, participate in organized leagues and pickup games to play sports such as basketball, tennis, baseball, football and soccer. However, Americans frequently utilize the healthcare system for treatment of injuries resulting from everyday activities such as sports. Nearly 2 million people every year, many of whom are otherwise healthy, suffer sports-related injuries and receive treatment in emergency departments. Some sports-related injuries, such as sprained ankles, may be relatively minor, while others, such as head or neck injuries, can be quite serious.

First Aid

First aid refers to medical attention that is usually administered immediately after the injury occurs and at the location where it occurred.

It often consists of a one-time, short-term treatment and requires little technology or training to administer.

First aid can include:

- cleaning minor cuts, scrapes, or scratches;

About This Chapter: Text in this chapter begins with excerpts from "Common Sports Injuries: Incidence And Average Charges" U.S Department of Health and Human Services (HHS), March 17, 2014; Text under the heading "First Aid" is excerpted from "Safety And Health Topics—Medical And First Aid," Occupational Safety and Health Administration (OSHA), May 1, 2005. Reviewed July 2017; Text under the heading "The Most Common Musculoskeletal Sports-Related Injuries" is excerpted from "Preventing Musculoskeletal Sports Injuries In Youth: A Guide For Parents," National Institute of Arthritis and Musculoskeletal and Skin Diseases (NIAMS), September 2016; Text under the heading "What Should I Do If I Suffer An Injury?" is excerpted from "Handout On Health: Sports Injuries," National Institute of Arthritis and Musculoskeletal and Skin Diseases (NIAMS), February 2016.

- treating a minor burn;

- applying bandages and dressings;

- the use of nonprescription medicine;

- draining blisters;

- removing debris from the eyes;

- massage; and

- drinking fluids to relieve heat stress.

The Most Common Musculoskeletal Sports-Related Injuries

Although sports injuries can range from scrapes and bruises to serious brain and spinal cord injuries, most fall somewhere between the two extremes. Here are some of the more common types of injuries.

Sprains And Strains

A sprain is an injury to a ligament, one of the bands of tough, fibrous tissue that connects two or more bones at a joint and prevents excessive movement of the joint. An ankle sprain is the most common athletic injury.

A strain is an injury to either a muscle or a tendon. A muscle is a tissue composed of bundles of specialized cells that, when stimulated by nerve messages contract and produce movement. A tendon is a tough, fibrous cord of tissue that connects muscle to bone. Muscles in any part of the body can be injured.

Growth Plate Injuries

In some sports accidents and injuries, the growth plate may be injured. The growth plate is the area of developing tissues at the end of the long bones in growing children and adolescents. When growth is complete, sometime during adolescence, the growth plate is replaced by solid bone. The long bones in the body include:

- the long bones of the hand and fingers (metacarpals and phalanges)

- both bones of the forearm (radius and ulna)

- the bone of the upper leg (femur)

- the lower leg bones (tibia and fibula)

- the foot bones (metatarsals and phalanges)

If any of these areas becomes injured, it's important to seek professional help from an orthopaedic surgeon, a doctor who specializes in bone injuries.

Repetitive Motion Injuries

Painful injuries such as stress fractures (a hairline fracture of the bone that has been subjected to repeated stress) and tendinitis (inflammation of a tendon) can occur from overuse of muscles and tendons. Some of these injuries don't always show up on X-rays, but they do cause pain and discomfort. The injured area usually responds to rest, ice, compression, and elevation (RICE). Other treatments can include crutches, cast immobilization, and physical therapy.

The Most Common Sports Injuries Are:

- Sprains and strains
- Knee injuries
- Swollen muscles
- Achilles tendon injuries
- Pain along the shin bone
- Fractures
- Dislocations

What Should I Do If I Suffer An Injury?

Whether an injury is acute or chronic, there is never a good reason to try to "work through" the pain of an injury. When you have pain from a particular movement or activity, STOP! Continuing the activity only causes further harm.

Some injuries require prompt medical attention, while others can be self-treated. Here's what you need to know about both types:

When To Seek Medical Treatment

You should call a health professional if:

- The injury causes severe pain, swelling, or numbness.

- You can't tolerate any weight on the area.

- The pain or dull ache of an old injury is accompanied by increased swelling or joint abnormality or instability.

When And How To Treat At Home

If you don't have any of the above symptoms, it's probably safe to treat the injury at home—at least at first. If pain or other symptoms worsen, it's best to check with your healthcare provider. Use the RICE method to relieve pain and inflammation and speed healing. Follow these four steps immediately after injury and continue for at least 48 hours.

- **Rest**. Reduce regular exercise or activities of daily living as needed. If you cannot put weight on an ankle or knee, crutches may help. If you use a cane or one crutch for an ankle injury, use it on the uninjured side to help you lean away and relieve weight on the injured ankle.

- **Ice**. Apply an ice pack to the injured area for 20 minutes at a time, four to eight times a day. A cold pack, ice bag, or plastic bag filled with crushed ice and wrapped in a towel can be used. To avoid cold injury and frostbite, do not apply the ice for more than 20 minutes. (Note: Do not use heat immediately after an injury. This tends to increase internal bleeding or swelling. Heat can be used later on to relieve muscle tension and promote relaxation.)

- **Compression**. Compression of the injured area may help reduce swelling. Compression can be achieved with elastic wraps, special boots, air casts, and splints. Ask your healthcare provider for advice on which one to use.

- **Elevation**. If possible, keep the injured ankle, knee, elbow, or wrist elevated on a pillow, above the level of the heart, to help decrease swelling.

Who Should I See For My Injury?

Although severe injuries will need to be seen immediately in an emergency room, particularly if they occur on the weekend or after office hours, most musculoskeletal sports injuries can be evaluated and, in many cases, treated by your primary healthcare provider.

Depending on your preference and the severity of your injury or the likelihood that your injury may cause ongoing, long-term problems, you may want to see, or have your primary healthcare professional refer you to, one of the following:

- An orthopaedic surgeon is a doctor specializing in the diagnosis and treatment of the musculoskeletal system, which includes bones, joints, ligaments, tendons, muscles, and nerves.

- A physical therapist/physiotherapist is a healthcare professional who can develop a rehabilitation program. Your primary care physician may refer you to a physical therapist after you begin to recover from your injury to help strengthen muscles and joints and prevent further injury.

How Are Sports Injuries Treated?

The Body's Healing Process

From the moment a bone breaks or a ligament tears, your body goes to work to repair the damage. Here's what happens at each stage of the healing process:

- **At the moment of injury**: Chemicals are released from damaged cells, triggering a process called inflammation. Blood vessels at the injury site become dilated; blood flow increases to carry nutrients to the site of tissue damage.

- **Within hours of injury**: White blood cells (leukocytes) travel down the bloodstream to the injury site where they begin to tear down and remove damaged tissue, allowing other specialized cells to start developing scar tissue.

- **Within days of injury**: Scar tissue is formed on the skin or inside the body. The amount of scarring may be proportional to the amount of swelling, inflammation, or bleeding within. In the next few weeks, the damaged area will regain a great deal of strength as scar tissue continues to form.

- **Within a month of injury**: Scar tissue may start to shrink, bringing damaged, torn, or separated tissues back together. However, it may be several months or more before the injury is completely healed.

(Source: "Handout On Health: Sports Injuries," National Institute of Arthritis and Musculoskeletal and Skin Diseases (NIAMS).)

Although using the RICE technique described previously can be helpful for any sports injury, RICE is often just a starting point. Here are some other treatments your doctor or other healthcare provider may administer, recommend, or prescribe to help your injury heal.

Nonsteroidal Anti-Inflammatory Drugs (NSAIDs)

The moment you are injured, chemicals are released from damaged tissue cells. This triggers the first stage of healing: inflammation. Inflammation causes tissues to become swollen, tender, and painful. Although inflammation is needed for healing, it can actually slow the healing process if left unchecked.

To reduce inflammation and pain, doctors and other healthcare providers often recommend taking an over-the-counter nonsteroidal anti-inflammatory drug (NSAID) such as aspirin, ibuprofen, or naproxen sodium. For more severe pain and inflammation, doctors may prescribe one of several dozen NSAIDs available in prescription strength.

Though not an NSAID, another commonly used OTC medication, acetaminophen, may relieve pain. It has no effect on inflammation, however.

Immobilization

Immobilization is a common treatment for musculoskeletal sports injuries that may be done immediately by a trainer or paramedic. Immobilization involves reducing movement in the area to prevent further damage. By enabling the blood supply to flow more directly to the injury (or the site of surgery to repair damage from an injury), immobilization reduces pain, swelling, and muscle spasm and helps the healing process begin. Following are some devices used for immobilization:

- Slings, to immobilize the upper body, including the arms and shoulders.

- Splints and casts, to support and protect injured bones and soft tissue. Casts can be made from plaster or fiberglass. Splints can be custom made or readymade. Standard splints come in a variety of shapes and sizes and have Velcro straps that make them easy to put on and take off or adjust. Splints generally offer less support and protection than a cast, and therefore may not always be a treatment option.

- Leg immobilizers, to keep the knee from bending after injury or surgery. Made from foam rubber covered with fabric, leg immobilizers enclose the entire leg, fastening with Velcro straps.

Surgery

In some cases, surgery is needed to repair torn connective tissues or to realign bones with compound fractures. The vast majority of musculoskeletal sports injuries, however, do not require surgery.

Rehabilitation (Exercise)

A key part of rehabilitation from sports injuries is a graduated exercise program designed to return the injured body part to a normal level of function.

With most injuries, early mobilization—getting the part moving as soon as possible—will speed healing. Generally, early mobilization starts with gentle range-of-motion exercises and then moves on to stretching and strengthening exercises when you can without increasing pain. For example, if you have a sprained ankle, you may be able to work on range of motion for the first day or two after the sprain by gently tracing letters with your big toe. Once your range of motion is fairly good, you can start doing gentle stretching and strengthening exercises. When you are ready, weights may be added to your exercise routine to further strengthen the injured area. The key is to avoid movement that causes pain.

As damaged tissue heals, scar tissue forms, which shrinks and brings torn or separated tissues back together. As a result, the injury site becomes tight or stiff, and damaged tissues are at risk of reinjury. That's why stretching and strengthening exercises are so important. You should continue to stretch the muscles daily and as the first part of your warm-up before exercising.

When planning your rehabilitation program with a healthcare professional, remember that progression is the key principle. Start with just a few exercises, do them often, and then gradually increase how much you do. A complete rehabilitation program should include exercises for flexibility, endurance, and strength; instruction in balance and proper body mechanics related to the sport; and a planned return to full participation.

Throughout the rehabilitation process, avoid painful activities and concentrate on those exercises that will improve function in the injured part. Don't resume your sport until you are sure you can stretch the injured tissues without any pain, swelling, or restricted movement, and monitor any other symptoms. When you do return to your sport, start slowly and gradually buildup to full participation.

Rest

Although it is important to get moving as soon as possible, you must also take time to rest following an injury. All injuries need time to heal; proper rest will help the process. Your healthcare professional can guide you regarding the proper balance between rest and rehabilitation.

Other Therapies

Other therapies used in rehabilitating sports injuries include:

- **Cold/cryotherapy**: Ice packs reduce inflammation by constricting blood vessels and limiting blood flow to the injured tissues. Cryotherapy eases pain by numbing the injured area. It is generally used for only the first 48 hours after injury.

- **Heat/thermotherapy**: Heat, in the form of hot compresses, heat lamps, or heating pads, causes the blood vessels to dilate and increase blood flow to the injury site. Increased blood flow aids the healing process by removing cell debris from damaged tissues and carrying healing nutrients to the injury site. Heat also helps to reduce pain. It should not be applied within the first 48 hours after an injury.

- **Ultrasound**: High-frequency sound waves produce deep heat that is applied directly to an injured area. Ultrasound stimulates blood flow to promote healing.

- **Massage**: Manual pressing, rubbing, and manipulation soothe tense muscles and increase blood flow to the injury site.

Most of these therapies are administered or supervised by a licensed healthcare professional.

Chapter 56

What Do Athletic Trainers Do?

Nature Of The Work

Athletic trainers specialize in preventing, diagnosing, and treating muscle and bone injuries and illnesses.

Duties

Athletic trainers typically do the following:

- Apply protective or injury-preventive devices, such as tape, bandages, and braces

- Recognize and evaluate injuries

- Provide first aid or emergency care

- Develop and carry out rehabilitation programs for injured athletes

- Plan and implement comprehensive programs to prevent injury and illness among athletes

- Perform administrative tasks, such as keeping records and writing reports on injuries and treatment programs

Athletic trainers work with people of all ages and all skill levels, from young children to soldiers and professional athletes. Athletic trainers are usually one of the first healthcare providers on the scene when injuries occur. They work under the direction of a licensed physician and with other healthcare providers, often discussing specific injuries and treatment options or evaluating and treating patients, as directed by a physician. Some athletic trainers meet with a team physician or consulting physician regularly.

About This Chapter: This chapter includes text excerpted from "Athletic Trainers," Bureau of Labor Statistics (BLS), U.S. Department of Labor (DOL), December 17, 2015.

An athletic trainer's administrative responsibilities may include regular meetings with an athletic director or another administrative officer to deal with budgets, purchasing, policy implementation, and other business-related issues. Athletic trainers plan athletic programs that are compliant with federal and state regulations, such as laws related to athlete concussions.

Athletic trainers should not be confused with fitness trainers and instructors, including personal trainers.

Work Environment

Athletic trainers held about 25,400 jobs in 2014. The largest employers of athletic trainers were as follows:

Table 56.1. Work Environment For Sports Instructors

Employers	Percent
Educational services; state, local, and private	37
Ambulatory healthcare services	26
Hospitals; state, local, and private	13
Fitness and recreational sports centers	11
Spectator sports	5

Many athletic trainers work in educational settings, such as colleges, universities, elementary schools, and secondary schools. Others work in hospitals, fitness centers, or physicians' offices, or for professional sports teams. Some athletic trainers work with military, with law enforcement, or with performing artists.

Athletic trainers may spend their time working outdoors on sports fields in all types of weather.

Work Schedules

Most athletic trainers work full time. Athletic trainers who work with teams during sporting events may work evenings or weekends and travel often.

Training And Other Qualifications

Athletic trainers need at least a bachelor's degree. Nearly all states require athletic trainers to have a license or certification; requirements vary by state.

Education

Athletic trainers need at least a bachelor's degree from an accredited college or university. Master's degree programs are also common. Degree programs have classroom and clinical components, including science and health-related courses, such as biology, anatomy, physiology, and nutrition.

The Commission on Accreditation of Athletic Training Education (CAATE) accredits athletic trainer programs, including postprofessional and residency athletic trainer programs.

High school students interested in postsecondary athletic training programs should take courses in anatomy, physiology, and physics.

Important Qualities

- **Compassion.** Athletic trainers work with athletes and patients who may be in considerable pain or discomfort. The trainers must be sympathetic while providing treatments.

- **Decision making skills.** Athletic trainers must be able to make informed clinical decisions that could affect the health or livelihood of patients.

- **Detail oriented.** Athletic trainers must record patients' progress accurately and ensure that they are receiving the appropriate treatments or practicing the correct fitness regimen.

- **Interpersonal skills.** Athletic trainers must have strong interpersonal skills in order to manage difficult situations. They must communicate well with others, including physicians, patients, athletes, coaches, and parents.

Licenses, Certifications, And Registrations

Nearly all states require athletic trainers to be licensed or certified; requirements vary by state. For specific requirements, contact the particular state's licensing or credentialing board or athletic trainer association.

The Board of Certification for the Athletic Trainer (BOC) offers the standard certification examination that most states use for licensing athletic trainers. Certification requires graduating from a CAATE-accredited program and completing the BOC exam. To maintain certification, athletic trainers must adhere to the BOC Standards of Practice and Disciplinary Process and take continuing education courses.

Advancement

Assistant athletic trainers may become head athletic trainers, athletic directors, or physician, hospital, or clinic practice administrators. In any of these positions, they will assume a management role. Athletic trainers working in colleges and universities may pursue an advanced degree to increase their advancement opportunities.

Chapter 57

Choosing A Doctor

When you choose a primary care doctor for yourself or a loved one, make sure to choose a doctor you can trust. A primary care doctor can:

- Help you stay healthy by recommending preventive services, like screening tests and shots

- Treat many health problems

- Refer you to a specialist when you need more help with a specific health issue

When you are choosing a doctor, look for someone who:

- Treats you with respect

- Listens to your opinions and concerns

- Encourages you to ask questions

- Explains things in ways you can understand

When you and your doctor work together as a team, you'll get better healthcare.

Ask For Recommendations From People You Know

Getting a reference from someone you know and trust is a great way to find a doctor.

- Ask friends, family members, neighbors, or coworkers if they have a doctor they like.

- If you are looking for a new doctor because yours is retiring or moving, ask your current doctor for a recommendation.

About This Chapter: This chapter includes text excerpted from "Choosing A Doctor: Quick Tips," Office of Disease Prevention and Health Promotion (ODPHP), U.S. Department of Health and Human Services (HHS), September 27, 2016.

Check With Your Insurance Company

If you have health insurance, you may need to choose from a list of doctors in their network (doctors that take you insurance plan). Some insurance plans may let you choose a doctor outside the network if you pay more of the cost.

- Call your insurance company and ask for a list of local doctors who take your insurance plan.

- Find out if your insurance company has a website you can use to search for a local doctor who sees people with your plan.

If you don't have health insurance, you'll have to pay for healthcare "out of pocket" (on your own). This can be very expensive.

Learn More About Your Top Choices

Make a list of the doctors you have in mind. Call their offices to learn more about them. The answers to the following questions may help you make the best decision.

Questions about the doctor:

- Is the doctor taking new patients?

- Is the doctor part of a group practice? Who are the other doctors?

- Who will see you if your doctor isn't available?

- Which hospital does the doctor use?

- If you have a medical condition, does the doctor have experience treating it?

Questions about the office:

- Do they offer evening or weekend appointments?

- What is the cancellation policy?

- How long will it take to get an appointment?

- How long do appointments usually last?

- Can you get lab work and X-rays done in the office?

- If you are more comfortable speaking in a language besides English, is there a doctor or nurse who speaks that language?

The First Appointment

After choosing a doctor, make your first appointment. This visit is a time for you to get to know the doctor and for the doctor to get to know you.

You will probably be asked to fill out a new-patient form. To help you, bring a list of your past medical problems and all the medicines you take. Include both prescription and over-the-counter drugs, even vitamins, supplements, and eye drops. Write down the dosage you take, such as 20 mg once a day. You might even put all your drugs in a bag and bring them with you to the appointment. Also, write down any drug allergies or serious drug reactions you've had. You will need to give all your drug information to the doctor to include in your medical record.

During the visit, take time to ask the doctor any questions you have about your health. You might want to write these questions down before your visit so you don't forget them. Some questions you may want to ask include:

- Will you give me written instructions about my care?
- May I bring a family member (spouse, daughter, or son) to my office visits?
- Are you willing to talk with my family about my condition if I give my permission?

During your first appointment, the doctor or nurse is likely to ask you questions about your current health and the medical history of your family. This information will also be added to your medical record.

After your first visit, think about if you felt comfortable and confident with this doctor. For example, were you at ease asking questions? Did the doctor clearly answer your questions? Were you treated with respect? Did you feel that your questions were considered thoughtfully? Did you feel the doctor hurried or did not address all your concerns? If you are still not sure the doctor is right for you, schedule a visit with one of the other doctors on your list.

Once you find a doctor you like, your job is not finished. Make sure to have your medical records sent to your new doctor. Your former doctor may charge you for mailing your records.

Remember that a good doctor-patient relationship is a partnership. Regular office visits and open communication with the doctor and office staff are important to maintaining this partnership, treating your medical problems effectively, and keeping you in good health.

(Source: "Choosing A Doctor," National Institute on Aging (NIA), National Institutes of Health (NIH).)

Think About Your Experience After The First Visit

Did the doctor and office staff:

- Make you feel comfortable during your appointment?
- Spend enough time with you?

- Give you a chance to ask questions?

- Answer your questions clearly?

If you answer "no" to any of these questions, you may want to keep looking.

Chapter 58

Guidelines For Medical Decision Making

Going to the doctor can be stressful, especially if you are sick or worried. You may also think that being a "good" patient means doing what your doctor tells you. But the truth is, staying quiet is not a good idea. By asking questions and understanding your treatment options, you can share in making decisions with your doctor and receive the best possible care.

What Is A Treatment Option, Anyway?

A treatment option is a medicine or therapy to treat your problem. A treatment option may be a pill, a shot, exercise, or an operation. It could even be a combination of things.

The process of fully exploring your options starts with asking your doctor questions about your diagnosis or condition. The next step is a full discussion about the available treatments—including the concerns you have about options and which options might be best for you.

It may seem okay to follow the first treatment your doctor suggests and then wait to see if it works. But if you take the time to talk to your doctor about all your treatment options, you may find one that works better for you.

About This Chapter: Text in this chapter begins with excerpts from "Explore Your Treatment Options: Why Explore Your Options," Agency for Healthcare Research and Quality (AHRQ), U.S. Department of Health and Human Services (HHS), October 6, 2011. Reviewed July 2017; Text under the heading "Next Steps After Your Diagnosis" is excerpted from "Next Steps After Your Diagnosis: Finding Information And Support," Agency for Healthcare Research and Quality (AHRQ), U.S. Department of Health and Human Services (HHS), July 2005. Reviewed July 2017; Text under the heading "Patient Rights" is excerpted from "Patient Rights," National Institutes of Health (NIH), August 31, 2016; Text under the heading "Informed Consent" is excerpted from "What Is Informed Consent?" Genetics Home Reference (GHR), National Institutes of Health (NIH), July 11, 2017.

How Can Knowing Your Treatment Options Improve Your Life?

You might feel better—not only about your health problem but also about your treatment choice and your part in decision making. Telling your doctor what is important to you can help you find the best medical care and improve your quality of life.

Talking about treatment options may help you find:

- A treatment or medical test that could work best for you.

- A treatment with fewer side effects.

- A treatment that's better for your budget.

- Better control over your healthcare.

Some people feel nervous about asking their doctor questions.

Remember: You know more about your body, your health, and what's important to you than anyone else. Don't be afraid to speak up.

Next Steps After Your Diagnosis

Five basic steps to help you cope with your diagnosis, make decisions, and get on with your life.

Step One: Take The Time You Need

A diagnosis can change your life in an instant. Like so many other people in your situation, you might be feeling one or more of the following emotions after getting your diagnosis:

- Afraid
- Alone
- Angry
- Anxious
- Ashamed
- Confused
- Depressed
- Helpless
- In denial

- Numb
- Overwhelmed
- Panicky
- Powerless
- Relieved (that you finally know what's wrong)
- Sad
- Shocked
- Stressed

It is perfectly normal to have these feelings. It is also normal, and very common, to have trouble taking in and understanding information after you receive the news—especially if the diagnosis was a surprise. And it can be even harder to make decisions about treating or managing your disease or condition.

Take time to make your decisions. No matter how the news of your diagnosis has affected you, do not rush into a decision. In most cases, you do not need to take action right away. Ask your doctor how much time you can safely take.

Taking the time you need to make decisions can help you:

- Feel less anxious and stressed.
- Avoid depression.
- Cope with your condition.
- Feel more in control of your situation.
- Play a key role in decisions about your treatment.

Step Two: Get The Support You Need

You do not have to go through it alone. Sometimes the emotional side of illness can be just as hard to deal with as the physical side. You may have fears or concerns. You may feel overwhelmed. No matter what your situation, having other people to turn to will help you know you are not alone.

Here are the kinds of support you might want to seek:

- Family and friends.
- Support or self-help groups.
- On-line support or self-help groups.
- Counselor or therapist.
- People like you.

Step Three: Talk With Your Doctor

Your doctor is your partner in healthcare. You probably have many questions about your disease or condition. The first person to ask is your doctor.

It is fine to seek more information from other sources; in fact, it is important to do so. But consider your doctor your partner in healthcare—someone who can discuss your situation with you, explain your options, and help you make decisions that are right for you.

It is not always easy to feel comfortable around doctors. But research has shown that good communication with your doctor can actually be good for your health. It can help you to:

- Feel more satisfied with the care you receive.

- Have better outcomes (end results), such as reduced pain and better recovery from symptoms.

Being an active member of your healthcare team also helps to reduce your chances of medical mistakes, and it helps you get high-quality care.

Of course, good communication is a two-way street. Here are some ways to help make the most of the time you spend with your doctor.

Prepare for your visit.

- Think about what you want to get out of your appointment. Write down all your questions and concerns.

- Prepare and bring to your doctor visit a list of all the medicines you take.

- Consider bringing along a trusted relative or friend. This person can help ask questions, take notes, and help you remember and understand everything once you leave the doctor's office.

Give information to your doctor.

- Do not wait to be asked.

- Tell your doctor everything he or she needs to know about your health—even the things that might make you feel embarrassed or uncomfortable.

- Tell your doctor how you are feeling—both physically and emotionally.

- Tell your doctor if you are feeling depressed or overwhelmed.

Get information from your doctor.

- Ask questions about anything that concerns you. Keep asking until you understand the answers. If you do not, your doctor may think you understand everything that is said.

- Ask your doctor to draw pictures if that will help you understand something.

- Take notes.

- Tape record your doctor visit, if that will be helpful to you. But first ask your doctor if this is okay.

- Ask your doctor to recommend resources such as websites, booklets, or tapes with more information about your disease or condition.

Do not hesitate to seek a second opinion.

A second opinion is when another doctor examines your medical records and gives his or her views about your condition and how it should be treated.

You might want a second opinion to:

- Be clear about what you have.

- Know all of your treatment choices.

- Have another doctor look at your choices with you.

It is not pushy or rude to want a second opinion. Most doctors will understand that you need more information before making important decisions about your health.

Check to see whether your health plan covers a second opinion. In some cases, health plans require second opinions.

Here are some ways to find a doctor for a second opinion:

- Ask your doctor. Request someone who does not work in the same office, because doctors who work together tend to share similar views.

- Contact your health plan or your local hospital, medical society, or medical school.

- Use the Doctor Finder on-line service of the American Medical Association (AMA) at www.ama-assn.org.

Get information about next steps.

- Get the results of any tests or procedures. Discuss the meaning of these results with your doctor.

- Make sure you understand what will happen if you need surgery.

- Talk with your doctor about which hospital is best for your healthcare needs.

Finally, if you are not satisfied with your doctor, you can do two things:

1. Talk with your doctor and try to work things out, and/or

2. Switch doctors, if you are able to. It is very important to feel confident about your care.

Ten Important Questions to Ask Your Doctor After a Diagnosis

It will help you understand your disease or condition, how it might be treated, and what you need to know and do before making treatment decisions.

1. What is the technical name of my disease or condition, and what does it mean in plain English?

2. What is my prognosis (outlook for the future)?

3. How soon do I need to make a decision about treatment?

4. Will I need any additional tests, and if so what kind and when?

5. What are my treatment options?

6. What are the pros and cons of my treatment options?

7. Is there a clinical trial (research study) that is right for me?

8. Now that I have this diagnosis, what changes will I need to make in my daily life?

9. What organizations do you recommend for support and information?

10. What resources (booklets, websites, audiotapes, videos, DVDs, etc.) do you recommend for further information?

Step Four: Seek Out Information

Now that you know your treatment options, you can learn which ones are backed up by the best scientific evidence. "Evidence-based" information—that is, information that is based on a careful review of the latest scientific findings in medical journals—can help you make decisions about the best possible treatments for you.

Evidence-based information comes from research on people like you.

Evidence-based information about treatments generally comes from two major types of scientific studies:

- Clinical trials are research studies on human volunteers to test new drugs or other treatments. Participants are randomly assigned to different treatment groups. Some get the research treatment, and others get a standard treatment or may be given a placebo (a medicine that has no effect), or no treatment. The results are compared to learn whether the new treatment is safe and effective.

- Outcomes research looks at the impact of treatments and other healthcare on health outcomes (end results) for patients and populations. End results include effects that people care about, such as changes in their quality of life.

Take advantage of the evidence-based information that is available.

Health information is everywhere—in books, newspapers, and magazines, and on the Internet, television, and radio. However, not all information is good information. Your best bets for sources of evidence-based information include the Federal Government, national nonprofit organizations, medical specialty groups, medical schools, and university medical centers.

Step Five: Decide On A Treatment Plan

At this point, you have learned about your disease or condition and how it can be treated or managed. Your information may have come from the following sources:

- Your doctor.

- Second opinions from one or more other doctors.

- Other people who are or were in the same situation as you.

- Information sources such as websites, health or medical libraries, and nonprofit groups.

Patient Rights

As a patient, you have certain rights. Some are guaranteed by federal law, such as the right to get a copy of your medical records, and the right to keep them private. Many states have additional laws protecting patients, and healthcare facilities often have a patient bill of rights.

An important patient right is informed consent. This means that if you need a treatment, your healthcare provider must give you the information you need to make a decision.

Many hospitals have patient advocates who can help you if you have problems. Many states have an ombudsman office for problems with long-term care. Your state's department of health may also be able to help.

Informed Consent

Informed consent can only be given by adults who are competent to make medical decisions for themselves. For children and others who are unable to make their own medical decisions (such as people with impaired mental status), informed consent can be given by a parent, guardian, or other person legally responsible for making decisions on that person's behalf.

Chapter 59

Return To Play

A question that is often asked by injured athletes and their coaches and parents is, "When can sports resume?" Return to play (RTP) decisions are frequently controversial, and there can be differences of opinion between healthcare providers and others. But there are specific policies in place for certain sports and specific injuries that can help guide athletes in making the right decision on RTP. The process has to be clearly understood by the athletes and families so that they can work with their doctor and physical therapist in RTP decisions.

Injuries mostly occur at the vulnerable structures of the body, like ligaments, tendons, and bones. If the athlete returns to the sport before full recovery, the injury can easily become worse. A mild sprain could become severe; a stress fracture can turn into a complete fracture; or a mild concussion might result in secondary brain injury or even death.

Recovery From Sports Injuries

An athlete should follow a seven-step treatment and rehabilitation program before returning to play:

1. **Encourage complete healing.** Healing time can vary depending on the site, severity, and type of injury. A ligament sprain may take 2 to 4 weeks to heal, whereas a leg fracture will take 8 to 12 weeks. Swelling, if any, has to come down fully. During this time, an athlete can keep him- or herself fit by doing some exercises (working the uninjured limb) or activities like swimming that will not put stress on the injured area. This should be done under the guidance of a physician or a physical therapist.

"Return To Play," © 2017 Omnigraphics. Reviewed July 2017.

2. **Restore pain-free full range of motion.** For most of the healing time, the injured part will be immobilized using a splint or a cast, which can result in reduced range of motion in the joint or muscle. Before returning to play, the athlete should achieve full pain-free range in the joint by doing range-of-motion exercises prescribed by the physical therapist. A good rule to follow: no return to sports if there is any limited motion in a joint.

3. **Regain muscle strength.** Due to the rest and immobilization following injury, the muscles around the injured part will weaken. This reduction in muscle strength needs to be improved before returning to play. The trainer or physical therapist will prescribe progressive resistance exercises for the gradual return of optimal muscle strength required for the sport.

4. **Regain normal stride.** There should be no limping present with running and walking before returning to play. If present, the cause needs to reassessed and managed.

5. **Regain endurance.** Athletes can continue general conditioning exercises with cross-training during the recovery phase. Using an alternative exercise allows maintenance of good cardiovascular fitness while not interfering with the healing process. Activities like swimming, running in water, biking, and rowing are excellent alternative exercises to help maintain endurance.

6. **Regain sport-specific skills.** The athlete should be able to perform the specific actions required for the sport effectively. The agility, balance, and flexibility required must be fully restored, both to ensure performance and to reduce the chance of re-injury. For example, retraining a knee injury in football should involve the ability to run, stop, change directions, and jump.

7. **Regain confidence.** When an injury keeps an athlete out of competition, it can result in a lot of psychological stress. The athlete needs to work to regain full confidence in his or her performance levels. Returning to play too soon may increase the risk of re-injury, new injury, depression, or poor performance.

Working closely with sports medicine experts can help ensure that the injured athlete recovers fully by following the program advised by them. Even though there will be tremendous pressure on the athlete to resume as soon as possible, his or her health and safety must be given top priority. Therefore, a systematic recovery protocol has to be strictly followed every day, at all levels of play, from recreational players to elite athletes.

Psychological Factors In Successful Return To Sport After Injury

A great deal of scientific evidence proves that psychological factors play a major role in an injured athlete's successful return to competition. This needs to be taken into consideration during injury rehabilitation, so that the athlete stays calm, focused, and motivated before returning to play.

The following are examples of some of the psychological factors that can affect an injured athlete:

- **Emotions shift over time.** As rehabilitation protocols progress, the athlete feels more positive (confidence and readiness) with lessened negative emotions associated with the initial injury, such as anger, depression, and anxiety.

- **Positive psychological response.** An athlete's ability to cope with the stress of injury greatly influences recovery and progression through the rehab program. Staying motivated is crucial, and a positive psychological response is associated with faster return to play after injury.

- **Negative psychological response.** If an athlete has a negative outlook on the injury and rehab, the chances of returning to sports can be decreased, and the risk of re-injury is higher if he or she does return. A negative psychological response usually results in a poor outcome.

- **Fear.** This can remain a noticeable emotion at the time athletes return to play. But there have been reports of athletes who have successfully returned to sports describing an associated dissipation of fear by actually testing the injured body part through returning to play.

- **External pressures.** There can be considerable pressure on an injured athlete to return too soon. The athlete feels pressured to maintain his or her spot on the team and to avoid letting the team and the coach down. When an athlete yields to this pressure and returns to sports prematurely, he or she may subsequently increase the risk of re-injury.

Recommendations

The following recommendations can further help ensure that athletes are fully prepared to return to play following an injury:

- **Psychological screening.** During rehab, proper screening of athletes needs to be carried out to identify the risk of developing negative psychological responses. Strategies should be developed to address such issues as fear, lack of confidence, and motivation.

- **Performance expectations.** Realistic performance goals should be set. Visual imagery methods can be used during the entire rehab process to build confidence, self-esteem, and a sense of competence.

- **Support.** There has to be constant support from coaches, teammates, parents, and others so that athletes do not perceive the external pressure to return to play too soon.

Psychological readiness usually increases as athletes progress through the rehabilitation process. However, if an athlete's psychological readiness before competition is low, waiting a little longer before returning to the playing field may be the safest course of action.

References

1. "When Is An Athlete Ready To Return To Play?" American Academy of Pediatrics (AAP), November 21, 2015.

2. "Return To Play After Sports Injury," Momsteam.com, n.d.

3. Onate, James A., PhD, ATC, and John Black, J.D. "Return-To-Participation Considerations Following Sports Injury," National Federation of State High School Associations, November 10, 2015.

Chapter 60

Sports Injuries And Arthritis: Understanding The Connection

Osteoarthritis And Sports Injury[1]

Osteoarthritis (OA) generally appears late in life, after decades of wear and tear and physiological responses. Joint trauma related to sports or other types of injury, for example, causes acute joint inflammation, cartilage damage, and significant increase in long-term risk for the development of osteoarthritis. However, how these injuries predispose patients to osteoarthritis is unclear. Treatment goals following traumatic joint injuries are: improvement of symptoms and function; restoration of structure; and prevention of osteoarthritis development and progression. Repairs of ligament and meniscal injuries are well-established procedures and usually restore joint function. However, they do not prevent the later (5–15 years) development of joint degeneration in 50–60 percent of patients. Studies focusing on joint changes immediately after injury offer opportunities to examine events leading to posttraumatic osteoarthritis (PTOA) and to discern what constitutes a pathologic versus a healthy healing pathway. They also may provide insights into the extent to which injuries contribute to late-onset osteoarthritis.

About This Chapter: This chapter includes text excerpted from documents published by two public domain sources. Text under the headings marked 1 are excerpted from "Meeting On Post-Traumatic Osteoarthritis (PTOA)," National Institute of Arthritis and Musculoskeletal and Skin Diseases (NIAMS), June 28, 2010. Reviewed July 2017; Text under headings marked 2 are excerpted from "Post-Injury Response Could Be Key Step In Osteoarthritis Development," National Institute of Arthritis and Musculoskeletal and Skin Diseases (NIAMS), May 2012. Reviewed July 2017.

> **Osteoarthritis By The Numbers**
> - 27 million Americans with OA
> - 632,000 joint replacements due to OA each year
> - 11.1 million outpatient visits for OA
> - $13.2 billion spent on job-related OA
>
> *(Source: "A National Public Health Agenda For Osteoarthritis," Centers for Disease Control and Prevention (CDC).)*

State Of The Science[1]

Although surgical approaches to reattach torn ligaments, repair damaged menisci, and reassemble fragmented bones have become increasingly sophisticated, the improvements have not reduced the incidence of PTOA. While many researchers continue to explore strategies for restoring joint structure and biomechanical function, others are investigating pathological changes and natural healing processes that occur on cellular and molecular levels following injury.

Disease manifestations also vary. Some people may develop PTOA quickly, while the disease may progress more slowly in others. Studying the 40–50 percent of people who experience joint trauma but do not develop PTOA should provide insights into the behaviors (e.g., post-injury exercise), genetic factors, and molecular mechanisms that foster healing or protect joints. Anatomical differences between male and female joints, joints at various ages, and differences in joint integrity due to previous damage also may influence response to injury and progression of PTOA. Additionally, premature return to physical activity and subsequent re-injury appear to be triggers for earlier development of disease.

Post-Injury Response Could Be Key Step In Osteoarthritis Development[2]

The study, conducted in the laboratory of William Robinson, M.D., Ph.D., at Stanford University, found that a pathway called the complement system, which is a major component of the innate immune system, is critical to the development of OA. Through analyses of joint tissue and joint fluid from individuals with OA, they found that expression and activation of complement is abnormally high in people with OA. The innate immune system is designed to protect the body from harmful invaders such as viruses and bacteria. When cartilage is injured, the researchers found, the complement system is activated, leading to inflammation directed against the body's own tissues.

Current treatment for OA is primarily limited to relieving symptoms and replacing joints that are too damaged to function well, says Dr. Holers. However, this new research suggests that by giving an agent to block the complement system soon after an injury occurs, doctors may be able to prevent the subsequent occurrence of OA.

Prevention And Treatment[1]

The ability to observe changes in cell function and cartilage structure in intact joints could allow researchers to develop new hypotheses about the biochemistry underlying PTOA, and uncover biomarkers that will identify people who are at greatest risk of developing PTOA. Considering a broad spectrum of possible molecular markers would widen the community's perspective on PTOA and elucidate the roles of cell damage in this process.

Some data suggest that trauma alters the lubricating properties of synovial fluid. While viscosupplementation, such as injections of hyaluronic acid, may appear to improve joint function, at least in the short-term, evidence supporting the practice is inconclusive. Studies of synovial fluid physiology and response to injury may reveal additional compounds, such as lubricin-like molecules or selected microRNAs, that could interact with cartilage and chondrocytes to facilitate healing or prevent further damage.

Other potential treatments include intraarticular injections or oral administration of antioxidants, caspase inhibitors, and nitric oxide mediators. Injectable gene therapy approaches are being tested in small animal models. Participants repeatedly noted that the effects of injectable or oral therapies are likely to be modest, and several approaches may need to be combined to prevent PTOA by targeting multiple pathways.

The timing of interventions is also likely to be important. Caspase inhibitors, which prevent apoptosis, are being studied as an initial treatment for injuries. Osteochondral grafting of visibly damaged cartilage currently is an option for some patients, but is most effective if done before PTOA becomes severe. Participants speculated that when effective preventive therapies are available and clinicians can predict which patients are likely to develop PTOA, the treatment paradigm will encourage immediate evaluation and medical care.

Patient behavior following an injury also remains an uncontrolled variable that may influence PTOA. Many patients adapt their biomechanics to avoid pain, but inadvertently adopt unhealthy movement patterns that may increase their risk of joint degradation. Some adaptations are so subtle that only sophisticated laboratory tools can alert clinicians that additional physical therapy is needed. Researchers also were interested in understanding the optimal level and type of physical activity during recovery. Because muscle strength is an important aspect of joint mechanics, physical therapy regimens that maintain or restore muscle function while allowing the injured cartilage and connective tissue to recover could delay PTOA.

Part Five
If You Need More Information

Chapter 61

Resources For More Information About Traumatic And Chronic Sports-Related Injuries

Academy for Sports Dentistry
118 Faye St. P.O. Box 364
Farmersville, IL 62533
Toll-Free: 800-273-1788
Fax: 217-227-3438
Website: www.academyforsportsdentistry.org
E-mail: info@academyforsportsdentistry.org

American Academy of Orthopaedic Surgeons (AAOS)
9400 W. Higgins Rd.
Rosemont, IL 60018
Phone: 847-823-7186
Fax: 847-823-8125
Website: www.aaos.org
E-mail: custserv@aaos.org

About This Chapter: Resources in this chapter were compiled from several sources deemed reliable; all contact information was verified and updated in July 2017.

American Academy of Otolaryngology—Head and Neck Surgery (AAO-HNSF)

1650 Diagonal Rd.
Alexandria, VA 22314
Phone: 703-836-4444
Website: www.entnet.org

American Academy of Pediatrics (AAP)

141 N.W. Pt. Blvd.
Elk Grove Village, IL 60007-1098
Phone: 847-434-4000
Fax: 847-434-8000
Website: www.aap.org

American Academy of Physical Medicine and Rehabilitation (AAPM&R)

9700 W. Bryn Mawr Ave.
Ste. 200
Rosemont, IL 60018
Phone: 847-737-6000
Fax: 847-737-6001
Website: www.aapmr.org
E-mail: info@aapmr.org

American Academy of Podiatric Sports Medicine (AAPSM)

3121 N.E. 26th St.
Ocala, FL 34470
Phone: 352-620-8562
Website: www.aapsm.org
E-mail: info@aapsm.org

American Association of Endodontists (AAE)

211 E. Chicago Ave.
Ste. 1100
Chicago, IL 60611-2691
Toll-Free: 800-872-3636
Phone: 312-266-7255
Toll-Free Fax: 800-451-9020
Fax: 312-266-9867
Website: www.aae.org
E-mail: info@aae.org

American Association of Neurological Surgeons (AANS)

5550 Meadowbrook Dr.
Rolling Meadows, IL 60008-3852
Toll-Free: 888-566-AANS (888-566-2267)
Phone: 847-378-0500
Fax: 847-378-0600
Website: www.aans.org
E-mail: info@aans.org

American Chiropractic Association (ACA)

1701 Clarendon Blvd.
Ste. 200
Arlington, VA 22209
Phone: 703-276-8800
Fax: 703-243-2593
Website: www.acatoday.org
E-mail: memberinfo@acatoday.org

American Chiropractic Association (ACA) Sports Council

2405 W. Main St.
Ste. 8
Bozeman, MT 59718
Phone: 623-694-2638
Website: www.acasc.org

American College of Foot and Ankle Surgeons (ACFAS)

8725 W. Higgins Rd.
Ste. 555
Chicago, IL 60631
Toll-Free: 800-421-2237
Phone: 773-693-9300
Fax: 773-693-9304
Website: www.acfas.org
E-mail: info@acfas.org

American College of Sports Medicine (ACSM)

401 W. Michigan St.
Indianapolis, IN 46202-3233
Phone: 317-637-9200
Fax: 317-634-7817
Website: www.acsm.org

American Medical Athletic Association (AMAA)

4405 E.W. Hwy
Ste. 405
Bethesda, MD 20814
Toll-Free: 800-776-2732
Phone: 301-913-9517
Fax: 301-913-9520
Website: www.amaasportsmed.org
E-mail: aama@americanrunning.org

American Medical Society for Sports Medicine (AMSSM)

4000 W. 114th St., Ste. 100
Leawood, KS 66211
Phone: 913-327-1415
Fax: 913-327-1491
Website: www.amssm.org

American Orthopaedic Foot and Ankle Society (AOFAS)

9400 W. Higgins Rd., Ste. 220
Rosemont, IL 60018
Toll-Free: 800-235-4855
Phone: 847-698-4654
Website: www.aofas.org
E-mail: PRCinfo@aofas.org

American Orthopaedic Society for Sports Medicine (AOSSM)

6300 N. River Rd.
Ste. 500
Rosemont, IL 60018
Toll-Free: 877-321-3500
Phone: 847-292-4900
Fax: 847-292-4905
Website: www.sportsmed.org
E-mail: info@aossm.org

American Osteopathic Academy of Sports Medicine (AOASM)

2424 American Ln.
Madison, WI 53704
Phone: 608-443-2477
Fax: 608-443-2474
Website: www.aoasm.org

American Osteopathic Association (AOA)

142 E. Ontario St.
Chicago, IL 60611-2864
Toll-Free: 888-62-MYAOA (888-626-9262)
Fax: 312-202-8202
Website: www.osteopathic.org
E-mail: crc@osteopathic.org

American Physical Therapy Association (APTA)

1111 N. Fairfax St.
Alexandria, VA 22314-1488
Toll-Free: 800-999-2782
Phone: 703-684-APTA (703-684-2782)
Fax: 703-684-7343
Website: www.apta.org

American Physiological Society (APS)

9650 Rockville Pike
Bethesda, MD 20814-3991
Phone: 301-634-7164
Fax: 301-634-7241
Website: www.the-aps.org

American Red Cross (ARC)

Website: www.redcross.org

American Shoulder and Elbow Surgeons (ASES)

9400 W. Higgins Rd.
Ste. 500
Rosemont, IL 60018
Phone: 847-698-1629
Fax: 847-268-9499
Website: www.ases-assn.org
E-mail: ases@aaos.org

American Society for Surgery of the Hand (ASSH)

822 W. Washington Blvd.
Chicago, IL 60607
Phone: (312) 880-1900
Website: www.assh.org
E-mail: info@assh.org

Ann & Robert H. Lurie Children's Hospital of Chicago
225 E. Chicago Ave.
Chicago, IL 60611
Toll-Free: 800-KIDS-DOC (800-543-7362)
Website: www.luriechildrens.org

Arthritis Foundation
1355 Peachtree St. N.E.
Atlanta, GA 30357-0669
Toll-Free: 800-283-7800
Phone: 404-872-7100
Website: www.arthritis.org

Brain Injury Association of America (BIAA)
1608 Spring Hill Rd.
Ste. 110
Vienna, VA 22182
Toll-Free: 800-444-6443 (Brain Injury Information Only)
Phone: 703-761-0750
Fax: 703-761-0755
Website: www.biausa.org

Bicycle Helmet Safety Institute (BHSI)
4611 Seventh St. S.
Arlington, VA 22204-1419
Phone: 703-486-0100
Website: www.bhsi.org
E-mail: info@helmets.org

Canadian Society for Exercise Physiology (CSEP)
18 Louisa St.
Ste. 370
Ottawa, ON K1R 6Y6
Phone: 877-651-3755
Fax: 613-234-3565
Website: www.csep.ca
E-mail: info@csep.ca

Children's Hospital Colorado

Anschutz Medical Campus
13123 E. 16th Ave.
Aurora, CO 80045
Toll-Free: 800-624-6553
Phone: 720-777-1234
Website: www.childrenscolorado.org

Christopher and Dana Reeve Foundation

636 Morris Turnpike, Ste. 3A
Short Hills, NJ 07078
Toll-Free: 800-225-0292
Phone: 973-379-2690
Website: www.christopherreeve.org

Coastal Physiotherapy & Sports Injury Clinic

123 Minnie St.
Southport, QLD 4215
Phone: (07)5-574-4303
Fax: 075-57271071
Website: www.coastalphysioclinic.com.au

Consumer Product Safety Commission (CPSC)

4330 E. W. Hwy
Bethesda, MD 20814
Toll-Free: 800-638-2772 (8:00 a.m. to 5:30 p.m. EST)
Phone: 301-504-7923 (General Information; Monday through Friday 8:00 a.m. to 4:30 p.m. EST)
Fax: 301-504-0124 and 301-504-0025
Website: www.cpsc.gov

Eunice Kennedy Shriver *National Institute of Child Health and Human Development (NICHD)*

P.O. Box 3006
Rockville, MD 20847
Phone: 301-496-5133
Toll-Free: 1-800-370-2943
TTY: 1-888-320-6942
Fax: 1-866-760-5947
E-mail: NICHDInformationResourceCenter@mail.nih.gov
Website: www.nichd.nih.gov

353

Gatorade Sports Science Institute (GSSI)

617 W. Main St.
Barrington, IL 60010
Toll-Free: 800-616-GSSI (800-616-4774)
Website: www.cu.pepsico.com

Hospital for Special Surgery (HSS)

535 E. 70th St.
New York, NY 10021
Phone: 212-606-1000
Website: www.hss.edu

Ian Tilmann Foundation

102 Timberview Dr.
Safety Harbor, FL 34695
Phone: 727-726-3435
Fax: 727-725-9286
Website: www.theiantilmannfoundation.org
E-mail: iantilmannfoundation@tampabay.rr.com

Institute for Arthroscopy and Sports Medicine (IASM)

2100 Webster St.,
Ste. 331
San Francisco, CA 94115
Phone: 415-923-0944
Fax: 415-923-5896
Website: www.iasm.com
E-mail: surgerycoordinator@iasm.com

MomsTeam.com

60 Thoreau St.
Ste. 288
Concord, MA 01742
Phone: 978-610-6265
Website: www.momsteam.com
E-mail: support@MomsTeam.com

National Academy of Sports Medicine (NASM)

1750 E. Northrop Blvd.
Ste. 200
Chandler, AZ 85286
Toll-Free: 800-460-6276
Phone: 602-383-1200
Fax: 480-656-3276
Website: www.nasm.org
E-mail: nasmcares@nasm.org

National Athletic Trainers Association (NATA)

1620 Valwood Pkwy
Ste. 115
Carrollton, TX 75006
Phone: 214-637-6282
Fax: 214-637-2206
Website: www.nata.org

National Eye Institute (NEI)

Information Center
31 Center Dr. MSC 2510
Bethesda, MD 20892-2510
Phone: 301-496-5248
Website: www.nei.nih.gov
E-mail: 2020@nei.nih.gov

National Center for Catastrophic Sport Injury Research (NCCSIR)

Department of Exercise & Sport Science
209 Fetzer Hall
CB# 8700
Chapel Hill, NC 27599-8700
Phone: 919-843-8357
Fax: 919-966-9143
Website: www.nccsir.unc.edu
E-mail: nccsir@unc.edu

National Center for Sports Safety (NCSS)

2229 1st Ave. S.
Birmingham, AL 35233
Toll-Free: 866-508-NCSS (866-508-6277)
Phone: 205-329-7535
Fax: 205-329-7526
Website: www.sportssafety.org
E-mail: info@SportsSafety.org

National Institute of Arthritis and Musculoskeletal and Skin Diseases (NIAMS)

National Institutes of Health (NIH)
1 AMS Cir.
Bethesda, MD 20892-3675
Toll-Free: 877-22-NIAMS (877-226-4267)
Phone: 301-495-4484
TTY: 301-565-2966
Fax: 301-718-6366
Website: www.niams.nih.gov
E-mail: NIAMSinfo@mail.nih.gov

Nationwide Children's Hospital

700 Children's Dr.
Columbus, OH 43205
Toll-Free: 800-792-8401
Phone: 614-722-2000
Website: www.nationwidechildrens.org/healthinfolibrary

Nicholas Institute of Sports Medicine and Athletic Trauma (NISMAT)

210 E. 64th St., Fifth Fl.
New York, NY 10028
Phone: 212-434-2700
Website: www.nismat.org
E-mail: info@nismat.org

NIH Osteoporosis and Related Bone Diseases—National Resource Center

2 AMS Cir.
Bethesda, MD 20892-3676
Toll-Free: 800-624-BONE (800-624-2663)
Phone: 202-223-0344
TTY: 202-466-4315
Fax: 202-293-2356
Website: www.bones.nih.gov
E-mail: NIHBoneInfo@mail.nih.gov

North American Spine Society (NASS)

7075 Veterans Blvd.
Burr Ridge, IL 60527
Toll-Free: 866-960-6277
Phone: 630-230-3600
Website: www.spine.org

Orthosports

47–49 Burwood Rd.
Concord NSW 2137
Website: www.orthosports.com.au
E-mail: education@orthosports.com.au

Prevent Blindness America

211 W. Wacker Dr.
Ste. 1700
Chicago, IL 60606
Toll-Free: 800-331-2020 (8:30 a.m. to 5:00 p.m. CST, Monday through Friday)

Prevent Sports Eye Injuries

211 W. Wacker Dr.
Ste. 1700
Chicago, IL 60606
Toll-Free: 800-331-2020
Website: www.preventblindness.org
E-mail: info@preventblindness.org

Safe Kids Canada
150 Eglinton Ave. E.
Ste. 300
Toronto, ON M4P 1E8
Toll-Free: 888-537-7777
Phone: 647-776-5100
Website: www.parachutecanada.org/safekidscanada
E-mail: info@parachutecanada.org

Safe Kids USA
1255 23rd St. N.W.
Ste. 400
Washington, D.C. 20037-1151
Phone: 202-662-0600
Website: www.safekids.org

Sport Medicine Australia
National Hockey Centre
196 Mouat St.
First Fl.
Lyneham 2602
Phone: 02-6247-5115
Fax: 02-6230-6676
Website: www.sma.org.au/contact-us

SportsMD Media
Phone: 203-689-6880
Website www.sportsmd.com
E-mail: contactus@sportsmd.com

SportsMed Web
Website: www.rice.edu/~jenky/sports

STOP (Sports Trauma and Overuse Prevention) Sports Injuries
W. Higgins Rd.
Ste. 300
Rosemont, IL 60018
Phone: 847-655-8660
Website: www.StopSportsInjuries.org
E-mail: info@stopsportsinjuries.org

University of Pittsburgh Medical Center (UPCM) Sports Medicine

200 Lothrop St.
Pittsburgh, PA 15213-2582
Toll-Free: 800-533-UPMC (800-533-8762)
Phone: 412-647-UPMC (412-647-8762)
Website: www.upmc.com

Chapter 62

Resources For More Information About Fitness And Exercise

Action for Healthy Kids

600 W. Van Buren St.
Ste. 720
Chicago, IL 60607
Toll-Free: 800-416-5136
Fax: 312-212-0098
Website: www.actionforhealthykids.org
E-mail: lcoleman@ActionforHealthyKids.org

Aerobics and Fitness Association of America (AFAA)

1750 E. Northrop Blvd.
Ste. 200
Chandler, AZ 85286-1744
Toll-Free: 800-446-2322
Website: www.afaa.com
E-mail: customerservice@afaa.com

About This Chapter: Resources in this chapter were compiled from several sources deemed reliable; all contact information was verified and updated in July 2017.

Amateur Athletic Union (AAU)

National Headquarters
P.O. Box 22409
Lake Buena Vista, FL 32830
Toll-Free: 800-AAU-4USA (800-228-4872)
Phone: 407-934-7200
Fax: 407-934-7242
Website: www.aausports.org

American Academy of Allergy, Asthma, and Immunology (AAAAI)

555 E. Wells St.
Ste. 1100
Milwaukee, WI 53202-3823
Phone: 414-272-6071
Website: www.aaaai.org

American Athletic Institute (AAI)

Website: www.americanathleticinstitute.org

American College of Allergy, Asthma, and Immunology (ACAAI)

P.O. Box 738
Saratoga Springs, NY 12866
Phone: 518-796-6337
Fax: 845-271-4136
Website: www.americanathleticinstitute.org

American Council on Exercise (ACE)

4851 Paramount Dr.
San Diego, CA 92123
Toll-Free: 888-825-3636
Phone: 858-576-6500
Fax: 858-576-6564
Website: www.acefitness.org
E-mail: support@acefitness.org

American Diabetes Association (ADA)

2451 Crystal Dr.
Ste. 900
Arlington, VA 22311
Toll-Free: 800-DIABETES (800-342-2383)
Website: www.diabetes.org
E-mail: askada@diabetes.org

American Heart Association (AHA)

7272 Greenville Ave.
Dallas, TX 75231
Toll-Free: 800-AHA-USA1 (800-242-8721)
Website: www.heart.org

American Lung Association

National Headquarters
55 W. Wacker Dr.
Ste. 1150
Chicago, IL 60601
Toll-Free: 800-LUNGUSA (800-548-8252)
Website: www.lung.org
E-mail: info@lung.org

American Running Association (ARA)

4405 E.W. Hwy,
Ste. 405
Bethesda, MD 20814
Phone: 800-776-2732 (ext. 13 or 12)
Fax: 301-913-9520
Website: www.americanrunning.org

Aquatic Exercise Association (AEA)

P.O. Box 1695
Brunswick, GA 31521-1695
Toll-Free: 888-232-9283
Website: www.aeawave.com

Asthma and Allergy Foundation of America (AAFA)
8201 Corporate Dr.
Ste. 1000
Landover, MD 20785
Toll-Free: 800-7-ASTHMA (800-727-8462)
Website: www.aafa.org
E-mail: info@aafa.org

Bone Builders Program Fights Osteoporosis
University of Arizona
4341 E. Bdwy.
Phoenix, AZ 85040-8807
Phone: 602-470-8086 ext. 332
Fax: 602-470-8092
Website: www.cals.arizona.edu
E-mail: shday@ag.arizona.edu

Center for Young Women's Health (CYWH)
333 Longwood Ave.
Fifth Fl.
Boston, MA 02115
Phone: 617-355-2994
Fax: 617-730-0186
Website: www.youngwomenshealth.org
E-mail: cywh@childrens.harvard.edu

Disabled Sports USA
451 Hungerford Dr.
Ste. 608
Rockville, MD 20850
Phone: 301-217-0960
Fax: 301-217-0968
Website: www.disabledsportsusa.org
E-mail: information@dsusa.org

HealthyWomen

P.O. Box 430
Red Bank, NJ 07701
Toll-Free: 877-986-9472
Phone: 732-530-3425
Fax: 732-865-7225
Website: www.healthywomen.org
E-mail: info@healthywomen.org

IDEA Health & Fitness Association

10190 Telesis Ct.
San Diego, CA 92121
Toll-Free: 800-999-4332 ext. 7
Phone: 858-535-8979 ext. 7
Fax: 619-344-0380
Website: www.ideafit.com
E-mail: contact@ideafit.com

International Fitness Association (IFA)

12472 Lake Underhill Rd.
Ste. 341
Orlando, FL 32828-7144
Toll-Free: 800-227-1976
Phone: 407-579-8610
Website: www.ifafitness.com

Kidshealth.org

Nemours Foundation
Website: www.kidshealth.org

LiveStrong

1655 26th St.
Santa Monica, CA 90404
Website: www.livestrong.com
E-mail: support@livestrong.com

National Alliance for Youth Sports (NAYS)

National Headquarters
2050 Vista Pkwy
W. Palm Beach, FL 33411
Toll-Free: 800-688-KIDS (800-688-5437)
Phone: 561-684-1141
Fax: 561-684-2546
Website: www.nays.org
E-mail: nays@nays.org

National Association for Health and Fitness (NAHF)

10 Kings Mill Ct.
Albany, NY 12205-3632
Phone: 518-456-1058
Fax: 716-851-4309
Website: www.physicalfitness.org
E-mail: aerobic2@aol.com

National Center on Health, Physical Activity and Disability (NCHPAD)

4000 Ridgeway Dr.
Birmingham, Alabama 35209
Toll-Free: 800-900-8086
Fax: 205-313-7475
Website: www.nchpad.org
E-mail: email@nchpad.org

National Coalition for Promoting Physical Activity (NCPPA)

1150 Connecticut Ave. N.W., Ste. 300
Washington, DC 20036
Website: www.ncppa.org
E-mail: ayanna@ncppa.org

National Collegiate Athletic Association (NCAA)

700 W. Washington St.
P.O. Box 6222
Indianapolis, Indiana 46206-6222
Phone: 317-917-6222
Fax: 317-917-6888
Website: www.ncaa.org

National Heart, Lung, and Blood Institute (NHLBI)

P.O. Box 30105
Bethesda, MD 20824-0105
Phone: 301-592-8573
Website: www.nhlbi.nih.gov
E-mail: nhlbiinfo@nhlbi.nih.gov

National Institute of Diabetes and Digestive and Kidney Diseases (NIDDK)

31 Center Dr. MSC 2560
Bldg. 31 Rm. 9A06
Bethesda, MD 20892-2560
Phone: 301-496-3583
Website: www.niddk.nih.gov

National Osteoporosis Foundation (NOF)

251 18th St. S.
Ste. 630
Arlington, VA 22202
Toll-Free: 800-231-4222
Website: www.nof.org
E-mail: info@nof.org

National Recreation and Park Association (NRPA)

22377 Belmont Ridge Rd.
Ashburn, VA 20148-4501
Toll-Free: 800-626-NRPA (800-626-6772)
Website: www.nrpa.org

National Strength and Conditioning Association (NSCA)

1885 Bob Johnson Dr.
Colorado Springs, CO 80906
Toll-Free: 800-815-6826
Phone: 719-632-6722
Fax: 719-632-6367
Website: www.nsca.com
E-mail: nsca@nsca.org

PE Central

2516 Blossom Trl W.
Blacksburg, VA 24060
Phone: 678-764-2536
Fax: 866-776-9170
Website: www.pecentral.org
E-mail: pec@pecentral.org

President's Council on Fitness, Sports & Nutrition (PCFSN)

1101 Wootton Pkwy
Ste. 560
Rockville, MD 20852
Phone: 240-276-9567
Fax: 240-276-9860
Website: www.fitness.gov
E-mail: fitness@hhs.gov

Right to Play International

134 W. 26th St.
Ste. 404
New York, NY 10001
Phone: 646-649-8280
Website: www.righttoplayusa.org
E-mail: info@righttoplayusa.com

Shape Up America!

P.O. Box 149
Clyde Park, MT 59018
Phone: 406-686-4844
Website: www.shapeup.org

Society of Health and Physical Educators (SHAPE America)

1900 Association Dr.
Reston, VA 20191-1598
Toll-Free: 800-213-7193
Fax: 703-476-9527
Website: www.shapeamerica.org

Sport Singapore

3 Stadium Dr.
Singapore 397630
Phone: 011-6500-5000
Fax: 011-6440-9205
Website: www.sportsingapore.gov.sg

Weight-Control Information Network (WIN)

1 WIN Way
Bethesda, MD 20892-3665
Toll-Free: 877-946-4627
Fax: 202-828-1028
Website: www.niddk.nih.gov
E-mail: win@info.niddk.nih.gov

Women's Sports Foundation (WSF)

Eisenhower Park
1899 Hempstead Turnpike Ste. 400
E. Meadow, NY 11554
Toll-Free: 800-227-3988
Phone: 516-542-4700
Fax: 516-542-0095
Website: www.womenssportsfoundation.org
E-mail: Info@WomensSportsFoundation.org

Index

Index

Page numbers that appear in *Italics* refer to tables or illustrations. Page numbers that have a small 'n' after the page number refer to citation information shown as Notes. Page numbers that appear in **Bold** refer to information contained in boxes within the chapters.

A

AAAAI *see* American Academy of Allergy, Asthma, and Immunology
AAFA *see* Asthma and Allergy Foundation of America
AAOS *see* American Academy of Orthopaedic Surgeons
"About Sports Eye Injury And Protective Eyewear" (NEI) 119n, 233n
abuse, defined 47
ACAAI *see* American College of Allergy, Asthma, and Immunology
Academy for Sports Dentistry, contact 347
Achilles tendon injuries
    described 225
    sports injuries 181
acromioclavicular joint (AC joint), defined **248**
acromion, defined **248**
ACSM *see* American College of Sports Medicine
Action for Healthy Kids, contact 361
acute injuries
    versus chronic injuries 182
    perineum 275
    spinal cord 245
    ulnar collateral ligament tears 266
adaptive devices, spinal cord injuries 245

addiction, anabolic steroids 59
adhesive capsulitis *see* frozen shoulder
aerobic exercise
    fitness 6
    knee problems 290
    progression 217
    see also endurance exercise
Aerobics and Fitness Association of America (AFAA), contact 361
Agency for Healthcare Research and Quality (AHRQ)
    publications
        bone fracture risks 201n
        broken hip 281n
        hip fracture treatment 281n
        sports injuries and kids 201n
        treatment guidelines 329n
        treatment options 329n
"Alcohol Screening And Brief Intervention For Youth—A Practitioner's Guide" (NIAAA) 61n
alcohol use
    athletes 61
    drowning 154
Amateur Athletic Union (AAU), contact 362
amenorrhea, female athlete triad 46
American Academy of Allergy, Asthma, and Immunology (AAAAI), contact 362